QUOTES
AMERICAN

THE POWER OF VITAMIN D...

"When I first started taking extra vitamin D, I had a lot of pain in my lower back and was on three Aleve™ a day. After 60 days, I'm off of all pain relievers and pain free."

- Delores

"I had quite a bit of pain in the back and all over. I used to take a lot of Anacin™ for back pain... now I can do a lot more...my housework, baking in the kitchen. I also have more strength when shopping."

- Lorraine

"Before I felt like I didn't want to live. I had steady pain, I couldn't lie in bed, I had to get up and walk around every two hours - like all of my muscles were tingling and cramping up. When I tried to stretch out, I cramped up to my knees. I can now sleep 6-7 hours and when I wake up, I feel great. Before my toes would be numb. Now I have my feet back. Before I had a constant backache like a toothache and it would pull in the right hip...but now it's so much better. I haven't had a pain or cramp in my legs since. I also discovered I can't handle dairy products and now drink soy."

- Liz

"I run a machine where we have to load blocks that weigh 200-300 lbs. and I have to swing them around and do a lot of lifting and twisting side to side. That's where my problems came from. I have lower back pain because of arthritis...kept me off of work for two weeks, I used drugs the doctor prescribed that threw me for a loop, they were very expensive and they made me real drowsy; made me want to sleep all the time and not do anything. And it didn't help the pain. The **Fountain of Youth Program** *is helping a lot. Now there's no more pain and I can move freely."*

- Mary

"I was on Aleve™ 2-3 times a day, but now I can truly say that I am pain free and not taking any Aleve™. My husband also had back and knee problems and he's much better."

- Doris

"I have degenerative arthritis in my right shoulder...the rotation is gone and the doctor wants to replace the total shoulder, but I'm too young for that. I was up to 12 tablets of painkillers a day just to be able to sleep. Now I'm down to only one or two...and I started taking extra vitamins C and D and omega-3 from flax and it's working."

- Matt

"My wife has fibromyalgia and the doctor gave her medication that made her feel loopy and when that didn't work, she took 5-6 Tylenol™ at a time just so she could sleep. Now she doesn't take any pain killers. She's never felt better since her accident 12 years ago."

- Bill

"My husband and I had both suffered from knee pain for a number of years. We began taking vitamin D3, and after only about two weeks, we both discovered that our knees felt a lot better. The **Fountain of Youth Program** *has totally eliminated my knee pain, and greatly reduced my husband's."*

- Viola

"I have been snowmobiling for years, and developed enough aches and pains, so that two years ago I had to give it up. Since I've been taking vitamin D, my aches and pains are gone, I have more energy, and I am looking forward to going snowmobiling again!"

- Scott

"Prior to following the **Fountain of Youth Program**, *I had pain in my knees and hip when walking the hills of my land. After using vitamin D regularly, the pain is gone – plus I have more energy."*

- Roger

"I have been taking vitamin D for about two months now and boy do I feel great! For many years I had experienced joint pain in my neck and shoulders but after a couple of weeks on the **Fountain of Youth Program**, *the pain is nearly gone (and so are the headaches too)!"*

- Leon

"I had bad 'tennis elbow' for a couple of years from repetitively swinging a hammer. Six weeks after taking vitamin D, it completely went away."

- Mike

"My lower back and left knee was bothering me for quite some time and the knuckles on my right hand had been stiff and hurting. I began taking glucosamine in 2004. I noticed some improvement in my knee, but it bothered me at night, so I never got a good night's rest. In June I started following the **Fountain of Youth Program***. By the end of July, my knee was much improved and my lower back was improving too. My right hand still was stiff at the knuckles. By the end of August, my knee didn't bother me at all. September I turned 84 years old. I've got more pep now. Mowing the lawn doesn't bother my knee! I had given up golf because of my knee and my back. I played a round lately, and I shot in the 40s for nine holes. My back still hurts when I bend over too long, but it recovers much more quickly than before. I can honestly say taking vitamin D has improved my health so that I can continue doing the things I love to do, and I don't have to ask for a lot of help."*

- John

" 'As a species, way back, we were bathed in sunshine, we never had any shortage of it,' Dr. Hollis said. Of course, this all changed as people became more civilized, spent more time indoors, began wearing clothes and, now, sunblock – which inhibits production of vitamin D."

- Nancy Stohs, Food Editor, Milwaukee Journal Sentinel

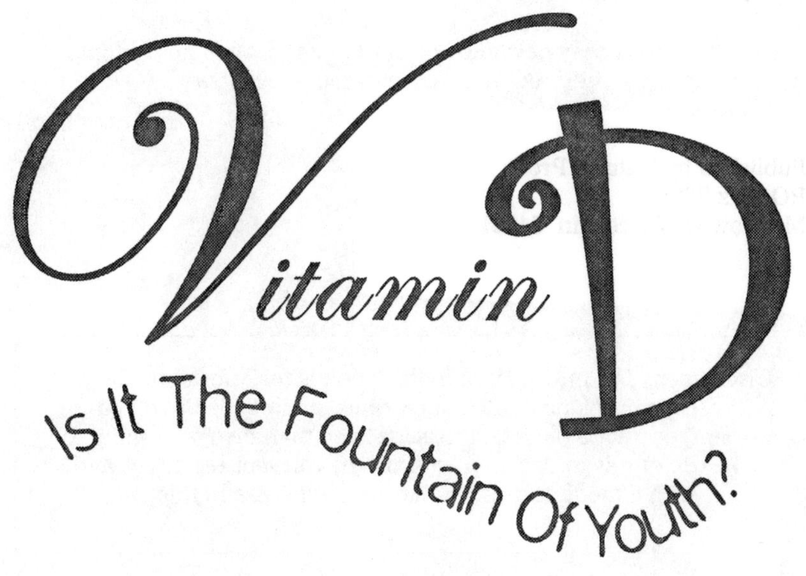

By Paul A. Stitt M.S., C.N.S.

Vitamin D - Fountain of Youth?

JMG ENTERPRISES
naturalpress@gmail.com
1631 S 17th St
Manitowoc WI 54220

Disclaimer: All information in this book is for informational purposes only. None of the suggestions are intended to diagnose, prevent, or treat a disease. It is suggested that anyone wishing to make use of this information consult the relevant resources and confer with a medical professional with expertise in this area.

Printed in the United States of America

Cover photo by Jerry Galas
Cover design by Christa Leonard, Lions Roar Studios

Substantial discounts on bulk quantities are available to corporations, professional associations, and other organizations.
For details contact Natural Press at 800-558-3535

ISBN 978-0-939956-11-1

ACKNOWLEDGEMENT

My heartfelt thanks to the many people who have made this book possible. First to my mother and father. Thanks to my teachers throughout many years in school for putting up with me. Thanks to all the media who have shown a lot of interest in my new ideas...Ron Zimmerman, WOMT talk show host, WGN-Radio, WOKY-TV, WTMJ-TV, Nancy Stohs at the *Milwaukee Journal* and writers at the *Minneapolis Star & Tribune, St. Paul Pioneer-Press, Chicago Tribune, Chicago Sun-Times, New York Times, Los Angeles Times, Atlanta Constitution* and many other newspapers.

I also wish to thank the Rotary Club, Optimists, Lions Club, Senior Centers and other service groups that have invited me to speak.

For helping to put this book together in record time, I wish to thank Jerry Galas and Kathy Kornelsen, my editors. Special kudos to Jerry and Bob who found ways to make vitamin D rich foods taste good. Most of all I wish to thank my fabulous wonderful wife, Barbara Reed Stitt, who has saved my life many times with her high energy and wonderful advice.

I also wish to thank the people who have been in desperate health and used this Fountain of Youth Program, proving that it really works. Thank you for buying this book. Please recommend it to your friends and those in media and politics who can spread the word about the miraculous benefits of vitamin D.

The very best to you and your loved ones,

Paul A. Stitt, Executive Director
Nutritional Resource Foundation

FOREWARD

What inspired me to write this book? I've been a student of nutrition and biochemistry for 40 years and have intensively studied vitamin D for the last three years; especially seeking answers to why my healthy son was diagnosed with osteoporosis at age 37.

I discovered there was no book published in the last 10 years that really explained the miraculous benefits of vitamin D. I am not a medical doctor. But I have learned that every disease should not be treated with an expensive, synthetic drug. Every "disease" has a biochemical cause and once you fix the cause of the problem, the "disease" will go away. This is what we biochemists were taught at the university. It really does work.

Testimonials given in the front of this book are in the words of real people who have used this complete, down-to-earth lifestyle program we call the **Fountain of Youth**. It can help you feel the best you've ever felt. It will work if you study and follow this practical program. For questions or comments, email me at *info@vitaminDinfo.org*.

Wishing you a safe and wonderful life,

Paul A. Stitt, M.S., Biochemist

INTRODUCTION

FINDING THE FOUNTAIN OF YOUTH

"Today, 10 million Americans have osteoporosis and another 34 million are at high risk. Each year, 1.5 million people have fractures and 20% will die within a year from their fractures. The number of hip fractures could triple in the next few decades. In 2002, fractures alone cost $18 billion dollars, and virtually all of them are preventable.""

- United States Surgeon General

The fountain of youth is not in some far-off, mysterious land, but available to those who sincerely seek to become free from chronic diseases and pain. Information on attaining your personal fountain of youth may be as close as your natural foods store.

What occurred to me in writing this book is that the agents capable of reducing the risk of osteoporosis, chronic pain, diabetes, cancer and other diseases will also make you feel better and younger. Conversely, agents that contribute to chronic diseases make you feel older, tired and depressed. In this book, we present an abundance of evidence that an adequate intake of vitamin D and improving your lifestyle will create your personal fountain of youth.

I know this to be true for myself after intensively studying vitamin D for over three years and personally experimenting with it for almost a year. As a trained biochemist, I know that vitamin D is by no means the only factor. A balanced diet of organically grown (if possible) fresh fruits, vegetables, whole grains, legumes, nuts, seeds, filtered water and exercise can help rejuvenate your health, *but the importance of additional vitamin D has been grossly overlooked for the last 50 years!*

Part of my knowledge comes from the experience my wife and I have gained from Natural Ovens Bakery, a company created in 1976. We bake highly fortified whole grain food products. We noticed that virtually all of the people who have worked for us at Natural Ovens for over 10 years look younger than their age, are not plagued with chronic diseases and are high energy people. Their health insurance costs are now going down each year. Most of Natural Ovens people are also good looking simply because their bodies feel good and this makes them feel happy. To us, this helps substantiate our belief that your body and your health can be no better than the quality of the food that you eat.

We formed the Nutritional Resource Foundation to educate and train people in the importance and health benefits of good nutrition for children and adults. Good nutrition can help prevent many degenerative diseases including obesity, bone problems, and diabetes as well as improve the academic ability and behavior of students in schools.

Ponce de Leon was first to seek the fountain of youth

Ponce de Leon went to Florida seeking the fountain of youth. He looked down expecting to find it on the ground. He should have been looking up at the sun. Sunshine gives us enough vitamin D if we expose our bodies to the mid-day sun for 20-30 minutes just three times a week, coupled with a good diet. All humans need a lot of vitamin D to feel really good. Aging accelerates if we don't get enough of it into our systems. Have you noticed that many people become depressed on cloudy winter days? In the absence of sunshine, adequate amounts of vitamin D will improve your mood.

Scientists have found that rapid aging can be caused by auto-immune diseases where the body starts destroying itself. One cell turns on another cell in our body, destroys it, and doesn't stop until all cells are destroyed. Vitamin D can stop that. Without D, the process just keeps going until we have no more energy or will to live. Vitamin D, along with other nutrients and antioxidants, can stop this process and make you feel years younger.

Drugs, pills, creams and lotions cannot reverse aging in the long run. They only help in the short-term.

A good healthy diet based on fresh fruits, vegetables and whole grains makes a huge difference in the long run. Avoid refined sugar, white flour, artificial flavors and colors and rich foods. Go for the foods that make you feel good and satisfied for hours. Good health is the best gift to give *yourself* at *any* time of the year!

The nature of disease

Understanding the nature of disease and pain requires diligence. Can you believe that the U.S. ranks only 27th in life expectancy? We are the biggest consumers of dairy products, but have the highest rate of osteoporosis. We undoubtedly have the most expensive medical care and the biggest economy, but we certainly miss the mark on being the healthiest.

In this book, we will discuss the real causes of chronic pain, osteoporosis, arthritis, diabetes, cancer and other diseases. Once you understand the basic causes, you'll be better equipped to manage your health and life. Choosing wisely, you may live to be 100 without aches, chronic pain or serious diseases. It's no fun growing old if you feel miserable.

We discovered our own fountain of youth

I was an old man at age 42, and that was 23 years ago. I was becoming obese, starting to lose mobility, my brain was not functioning very well, and I was unable to manage my anger. Luckily, I married Barbara Reed in 1982, who knew a lot about the fountain of youth. Even though she was 10 years my senior, I couldn't keep up with her physically, mentally or psychologically.

However, before we met, Barbara herself was an old lady in 1963 at age 33. She had skin cancer, diabetes, arthritis, periods of blacking out, petit mal epilepsy and early stages of menopause. Then she read the book *"Look Younger and Live Longer"* by Gaylord Hauser. It changed her life and after we came together in 1982, she went on to change my life.

A perfect combination: chocolate plus D

In 2003, I became intensely interested in the scientific literature on the many benefits of vitamin D. In early 2005, I began making dark chocolate clusters rich in vitamin D. We discovered that when you add enough nutrients to dark chocolate, they *actually discourage overindulging*. Since we started working with the chocolate – and doing lots of sampling – we have improved our health and fitness without gaining any weight.

Barbara has almost doubled her muscle strength. She no longer wears arch supports in her shoes as the muscles in her feet now support her arches. Her eyebrows and the roots of her hair are becoming dark instead of gray. I am no longer plagued by athlete's foot infections as I have been for 40 years and the roots of my hair are also coming in dark brown like when I was a kid. I couldn't even run when I was in high school; now I love to run. Plus, we both realized after a couple of months of eating the enriched chocolate clusters that we can now enjoy a glass of wine without getting a headache.

My wife and I feel we are experiencing our own fountain of youth here and now. We intend to keep working with the chocolates and turn it into a profit-making business that truly helps people feel the best they have ever felt in their life. If you want to know how we're doing, drop us a note at *info@vitaminDinfo.org*.

TABLE OF CONTENTS

CHAPTER ONE

D DEFICIENCY HAS A WORLDWIDE, LIFETIME EFFECT

"We absolutely have a huge problem with vitamin D deficiency."

- Dr. Bess Dawson-Hughes,
director of the Bone Metabolism Laboratory,
Tufts University

Vitamin D deficiency is rampant in America. Rickets, a disease of severe deficiency, is once again rearing its ugly head everywhere, including Wisconsin, the Dairy State. It's costing every American a great deal of pain and a lot of money for expensive medical treatment. Whenever people avoid the noonday sun, and avoid eating liver and fatty fish, they become more and more deficient. Chronic pain is the first sign of deficiency. 40% of our American workforce has chronic pain on a weekly basis. Surveys have shown that 70% of all Americans of every race, and from every walk of life, whether rich and poor, are deficient.

The impact of vitamin D deficiency begins at conception. Very early in pregnancy, D deficiency can increase the risk of type-I diabetes, and cause slow brain development, often contributing to a child being born with a lower IQ. During the first year of life, D deficiency also increases the risk of type-II diabetes, often leading to obesity. A mother-to-be who is vitamin D deficient can unwittingly contribute to her child's future health problems by giving birth to a child who could be destined to become overweight and a slow learner. Deficiency in the early years also leads to weak, brittle bones and increased risk of fractures from minor falls among children. In mid-life, the problem persists and often gets worse.

My son's accident launched me on a journey

At the age of 37, my son had a minor bicycle accident and broke his hip. Luckily, he went to a doctor who not only treated the fracture, but also looked for the underlying cause. The doctor found that my son had osteoporosis, despite the fact he ate a healthy diet every day of his life, including whole grain breads, plenty of fruits and vegetables and lots of dairy products (we lived on a dairy farm and I owned a cheese store, so he had plenty of calcium every day). How could my son have osteoporosis? Because, at that time, the best diet available was very deficient in vitamin D, and he grew up in Wisconsin, far north of the Mason Dixon line that almost guarantees a lack of the sunshine vitamin. The amount of vitamin D that doctors and dieticians recommend today is still woefully insufficient.

Researchers and FDA officials now recommend dramatically raising the recommended level of vitamin D in all diets to significantly more than the 200-600 unit recommendation that is still the official standard among practitioners. *That low recommendation level was based on the minimum amount of vitamin D thought to just prevent rickets.* Researchers now believe 40% of the young people in America are vitamin D deficient.

Vitamin D *deficiency* weakens white blood cells that fight infections and kill cells that can become cancerous. Harvard University researchers found that deficiency increases the risk of 27 different types of cancer by 30-40%; specifically colon, mammary, prostate and ovarian cancer. Deficiency also causes chronic bone and muscle pain. The University of Minnesota and the Mayo Clinic reported that 93% of the people with chronic pain have severe deficiency, whether they are young or old. Some 99% of the home-bound elderly are believed to be vitamin D deficient, as well as 42% of doctors in South Florida, where there is plenty of sunshine and opportunities to be outdoors.

Vitamin D deficiency is an epidemic

Vitamin D deficiency increases the risk of dying from heart disease by 25%, plus it leads to osteoporosis and humped-back shoulders in the aged. Here again, it first causes weak muscles and then frail bones. Weak muscles make it difficult for people to walk with confidence. They sway, lose their balance, fall and then, because of weak bones, they're more likely to fracture their hips, spines or other bones. If deficient, their bones don't heal well and a high percentage die from falls and fractures, especially here in my home city of Manitowoc, Wisconsin. Wisconsin ranks as one of five top states with the most deaths from falls and fractures, and Manitowoc County has the highest death rate from falls in the state. Over half the calls to paramedics involve people who have fallen and can't get up. Fear of death from falling is all too real for too many Americans.

You can do something about this problem by taking charge of your good health, instead of waiting for the government, your doctor or your pharmacist to do it for you. Stopping this epidemic can also be quite pleasurable. You can spend 30 minutes per day exposing 30% of your skin to noontime sun at least three times a week, or eat foods that are highly fortified with vitamin D. My journey to find the real truth behind the reason my son was diagnosed with osteoporosis has led me on a wild and amazing journey.

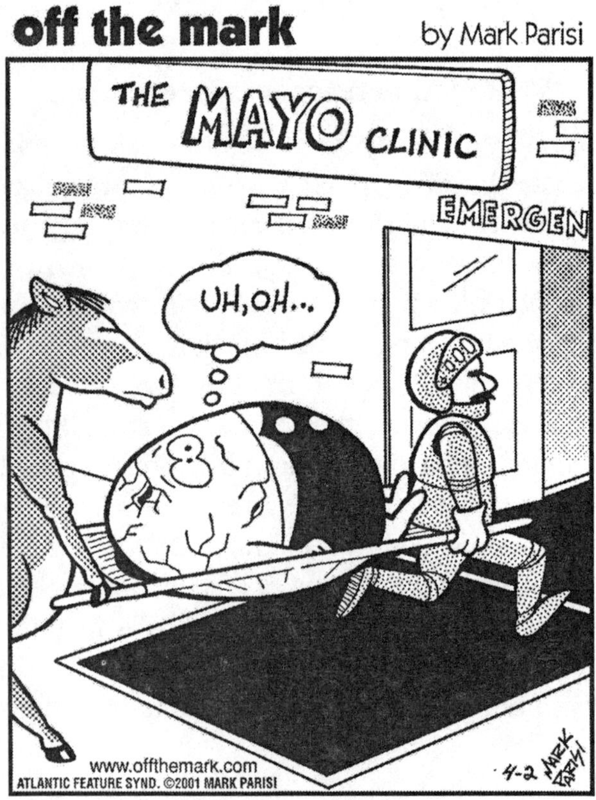

Cartoon copyrighted by Mark Parisi, printed with permission

CHAPTER TWO

NATIONAL LIBRARY OF MEDICINE HAS SHOCKING STATISTICS

> *"It is now recognized that most of the population in the United States is at a risk for vitamin D deficiency."*
>
> \- Dr. Michael Holick,
> Boston University Medical Center

- 32% of doctors and medical school students are vitamin D deficient
- 42% of the doctors in South Florida are D deficient
- 42% of otherwise healthy young adults in the U.S. are D deficient
- 40% of the U.S. population is vitamin D deficient
- 85% of African-American women of childbearing age are deficient
- 48% of young girls (9-11 years old) are vitamin D deficient
- Up to 90% of all hospital patients are deficient
- 76% of pregnant mothers are severely vitamin D deficient, causing widespread deficiencies in their unborn children, predisposing them to type-I diabetes, arthritis, multiple sclerosis and schizophrenia later in life. 81% of the children born to these mothers are deficient

- Up to 99% of nursing home patients are deficient
- 93% of Americans with chronic pain are vitamin D deficient
- 65% of the people in Chicago are vitamin D deficient (not enough sunshine)
- The major cause of osteoporosis and chronic pain is vitamin D deficiency and cannot be cured without adequate vitamin D

An April, 2000, clinical observation published in the *Archives of Internal Medicine* caught my attention. Dr. Anu Prabhala and her colleagues reported on the treatment of five patients confined to wheelchairs with severe weakness and fatigue. Blood tests revealed that all of the patients suffered from severe vitamin D deficiency. They received 50,000 IU of vitamin D per week by injection and they all became mobile within six weeks. How could such a situation exist? Many people are left in pain for their entire lives just for lack of the Sunshine Vitamin. I found this to be an unconscionable, common occurrence in hospitals and nursing homes all over the world. I found that you cannot change them. There is simply too much money to be made from weak, helpless people.

Vitamin D affects form/function of every body cell

Vitamin D from food or sunshine turns into the most important and powerful hormone in the human body. It determines whether your bones and muscles are strong and free of chronic pain. Without strong bones and muscles, it really doesn't matter if your heart ticks or not. If your body is full of chronic pain, you may wish that your heart would stop ticking.

- Vitamin D hormone arms your immune system to kill bacteria and viruses that are invading your body every minute of every hour you are alive. Why live if you can't stay healthy?

- Vitamin D hormone directs your immune system so that it doesn't attack your own body. Strange as it may seem, this is the basic cause of diabetes, arthritis and other auto-immune diseases.

- Vitamin D hormone directs your body's immune system to kill rogue cancer cells. Without enough vitamin D, cancer cells can spread in unhealthy bodies.

- Vitamin D hormone determines how much calcium your body absorbs from your food. If you don't have enough D, your body can only absorb about 20% of the calcium from your food. (The excess calcium then settles in joints or other points of stress within your body.) With enough D, your body can absorb and use about 80% of the calcium, assuming you have consumed enough magnesium and not too much phosphate from too many processed foods and soft drinks.

So the incredible news is that *Vitamin D affects every phase of human development, from the moment of conception to your final moment.* Scientists have found that women who conceive during the fall and winter have babies with lesser brain development than those conceived during longer days of sunlight. Newborns who do not receive adequate D have insulin receptors that are not very responsive to blood glucose levels, and tend to have wildly fluctuating blood sugar levels, which may cause them to overeat. Children born with very low levels of D can also develop rickets, which is another name for very weak and soft bones. Children born with sub-optimal levels of D develop weak bones that are easily broken from low impact. Without adequate levels of Vitamin D, a child may be subject to low impact fractures throughout his or her life.

Vitamin D and the immune system

White blood cells with inadequate levels of vitamin D are unable to attack and kill cancer cells. Vitamin D affects the functioning of liver, lung and kidney cells. Heart muscle cells that are low in Vitamin D are weak and unable to pump blood efficiently. Main muscles that are low in vitamin D are weak, causing people to sway and become unsteady on their feet. Fear of falls keeps people from exercising as much as they should. Bone cells without adequate D are porous and can break easily, sometimes from just normal walking. Brain cells that do not get enough vitamin D don't work very well and a person can end up depressed or schizophrenic. Kidneys, lung and pancreas that don't work well can lead to diabetes, tuberculosis and kidney disease. As you can see, vitamin D affects the form and function of every cell in the body!

History of vitamin D

Vitamin D was discovered by several researchers at the University of Wisconsin. They also noted that simply exposing the skin to sun could create this amazing vitamin. In 1914, Dr. E.V. McCollum discovered vitamin D in cod liver oil. Dr. Harry Steenbock in 1923 discovered that exposing milk to UV light created vitamin D in milk. Henry DeLuca, Neal Binkley, Mary Elliott, Marc Drezner and others continue the tradition of discovery today.

In the 1940s, Canadian-born dentist Weston A. Price published his masterpiece, *Nutrition and Physical Degeneration*. He noted that the diet of isolated, so-called "primitive" peoples contained "at least 10 times" the amount of "fat-soluble vitamins" as the standard American diet of his day. Dr. Price determined that it was the presence of plentiful amounts of fat-soluble vitamin D in the diet, along with balanced levels of calcium, phosphorus and other minerals that produced strong bones, a high immunity to tooth decay and resistance to the diseases common to non-industrialized groups. Dr. Price was considered a quack, but we now know that his research was ahead of the times.

Russian light boxes

In the 1950s, the Russians used light boxes to cure people of all sorts of diseases. The boxes were little 3-sided houses without roofs. After three weeks of treatment, many people were cured of cancer, arthritis, heart disease and many other ailments. In the 50s, I was just starting to study the connection between nutrition and health as a young man on my father's farm. I thought this treatment was total nonsense. Now that I know the mechanism and how it works, I realize this method made a *lot* of sense.

This was followed by an era of antibiotics and new drugs for every ailment. High tech became the "in thing," while the old methods that actually worked very well became "old fashioned." Why would a doctor want to prescribe a cheap, almost universal cure, when there was a different and expensive drug for every ailment? If one of the drugs caused a serious side effect, another could always be prescribed for that ailment.

Today, another Canadian researcher, Dr. Reinhold Vieth, argues convincingly that current vitamin D recommendations are woefully inadequate. The recommended dose of 200-400 international units (IU) barely prevents rickets in children, but doesn't come close to the optimal amount necessary for vibrant health. According to Dr. Vieth, the minimal daily requirement of vitamin D should be in the range of 2,000 to 4,000 IU from all sources, or 10 times the Recommended Daily Allowance (RDA). Dr. Vieth's research perfectly matches Dr. Price's observations 60 years ago.

Information overload: 38,000 articles

The number of articles published in peer-reviewed scientific literature is voluminous, and I have spent years studying them. **There are 38,000 articles in the National Library of medicine on vitamin D and 13,000,000 citations in Google.** It's very difficult to sort through all of the information, while separating out the articles written by many drug companies and the calcium industry touting their latest "discoveries."

The amount of tainted research published today is unbelievable, as the Vioxx™ trials have shown. The trials have brought out the idea that as many as 60,000 to 140,000 people have died of heart disease, simply because Merck may have covered up damaging information and did not allow it to get published. Even the prestigious *New England Journal of Medicine* is involved because they were not told all the facts about Vioxx™ in the articles that were published in their journal. Here are the number of articles I have found concerning vitamin D and various diseases.

Numbers of scientific articles published

D and heart disease and high blood pressure: 495

D and learning ability and brain development: 247

D and type I and perhaps type II diabetes: 229

D and obesity: 54

D and muscle strength: 499

D and bone density: 899

D and cancer: 2131

D and osteoporosis: 1133

D and fibromyalgia and multiple sclerosis: 60

D and arthritis/rheumatism: 164

D and tuberculosis: 82

D and chronic pain: 149

No one in the medical field can say this book is just my opinion. Look again at the number of papers written on various diseases. Even the FDA is jumping on this bandwagon. They have published numerous papers on how the lack of vitamin D leads to increased risk for cancer, diabetes, osteoporosis and autoimmune diseases, as you will see in a later chapter. Experts from the FDA have chaired many seminars on the need for all Americans and Canadians to increase their vitamin D intake.

off the mark
by Mark Parisi
BEFORE MY PHYSICAL, COULD YOU ASSURE ME THAT YOUR MEDICAL JOURNALS ARE MORE UP-TO-DATE THAN THE MAGAZINES IN THE WAITING AREA?
MARK PARISI
offthemark.com
©1992 MARK PARISI

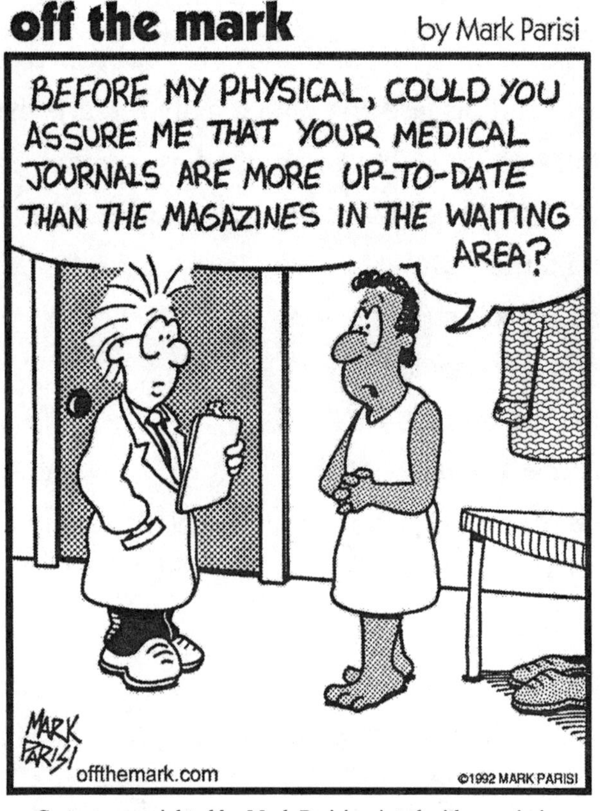

Cartoon copyrighted by Mark Parisi, printed with permission

CHAPTER THREE

BUILDING BETTER BONES BEGINS IN CHILDHOOD

"*It's pain that ages us, not years.*"

- Bonnie Prudden,
myotherapist and
author of *Pain Erasure*

Children born to women who maintain high vitamin D levels during pregnancy have bigger, stronger and more calcium-rich bones than any other children by age nine, a major protective factor against osteoporosis later in life. This new British study, reported in the prestigious *Lancet* medical journal, found that neither milk intake nor physical activity in childhood resulted in later bone strength. Another study showed that vitamin D supplements given to premature babies during their first year resulted in stronger bones by age 12. How can women get their maternal vitamin D levels up? The study identified only two ways: live in a place with a higher number of sunny days where the body is exposed to ultraviolet light, or consume vitamin D enriched food or vitamin supplements.

Unhealthy habits are putting today's children at risk for osteoporosis in greater numbers than ever before. The good news is that there is a way for you to protect your child, and yourself. Every time your child drinks soda, the groundwork is being laid for a dangerous bone disease. Fizzy and sugary soft drinks are laden with phosphate, which is a major binder of calcium that prevents calcium from being absorbed from food. This contributes to bone breakage and later, osteoporosis.

Drinking milk is no better, because cow's milk is also a major source of phosphate. So is processed meat and cheese. Adding phosphate to cheese makes it melt and flow more easily. Picture the soft cheese you see on an order of nachos and cheese. Extra high levels of salt, that leaches calcium out of bones, are also added for flavor. So what do young people live on? Lots of processed meats, cheeses, milk and sodas.

To make matters even worse, many young people avoid fresh fruit and vegetables, which are great sources of vitamin K. Vitamin K is absolutely essential for preventing osteoporosis. Yet, less than 5% of young people get the important five servings of each group daily. I learned this directly from the FDA's own in-house expert on osteoporosis, Dr. Mona Calvo, during a lecture she gave at a scientific meeting I attended.

Many children also lead a sedentary lifestyle, missing the bone-building benefits of vigorous exercise. Parents, as well, are reluctant to let their children go out and exercise for fear they might be harmed. These children are at risk of developing brittle bones and fractures decades down the road, and for developing osteoporosis at a younger age than ever before.

Osteoporosis actually a childhood disease

This is a problem every parent should be concerned about, says Leo Root, MD, author of *Beautiful Bones Without Hormones*, and professor of clinical orthopedics at

Weill Medical College of Cornell University in New York City. He adds: "Osteoporosis is actually a childhood disease that manifests itself later in life." This is just what my son discovered.

Vitamin D deficiency causes bones to become riddled with holes filled with fat, making them very susceptible to breaking. Weak bones can become broken bones, which, in turn, can cause deformity like the "widow's hump," chronic pain, and even disability. Osteoporosis can also hasten death; 20% of older people who suffer a broken hip die within a year.

Osteoporosis is not just your grandmother's problem. Although it strikes about eight million women, it also menaces two million men. Another 34 million Americans have low bone mass, yet most aren't even aware that there is an epidemic in the making, said Surgeon General Dr. Richard Carmona, who released the first-ever Surgeon General's report on osteoporosis in October, 2004. "You don't see TV shows like *Desperate Housewives* talking about osteoporosis, and it's not in the headlines like various movie stars. But by embracing prevention, we could save many thousands of lives and prevent millions from chronic pain and broken bones," he said.

"There's a new medical understanding of the best ways to protect ourselves and our children. Simple lifestyle changes can save your bones, which can save your life," stressed Dr. Root. "And it's never too soon, or too late, to take action."

The calcium disconnection

Contrary to popular belief, the skeleton isn't a rigid and unchanging structure made up only of calcium. Each year our bodies replace 20% of our bones' spongy tissue, which means that diet and activities at every age influence our health. Sections of bone develop micro fractures, creating gaps to be filled by new bone. The body then dissolves the ragged edge of the fracture, and with adequate nutrients like vitamin D, calcium, magnesium, B-12, and folic acid, it lays down a matrix to "weld" the bone back together.

Many drugs that treat osteoporosis actually prevent the body from dissolving the ragged edge of the micro fracture, causing the bone to maintain more density, while making it very vulnerable to breaks. One woman told me that while she was on several different osteoporosis drugs for five years, she had 20 fractures of various bones in her body. If she had consumed enough vitamin D and other essential nutrients, her bones would have healed and become very strong. Drugs alone just can't do it.

Think of your bones as a retirement fund: The more you deposit when you are young, the better off you will be in later years when you need to draw on your reserves. But most kids don't consume nearly enough nutrients, believing it's not cool to eat healthy foods. Not yet, at least.

There's a lot of debate about how much calcium is enough, and it's very easy to get too much. Too much prevents the absorption of other nutrients and it also prevents the conversion of messenger vitamin D into activated vitamin D. Here's the trick. With low D intake of less then 1,000 IU for a child, the body only absorbs about 20%

of the calcium it ingests. With adequate D, 2,000 IU or more per day for an adult, the body absorbs up to 80% of the calcium from food.

Since only about 20% of the young people in America get enough combined D from the sun and diet, it's easy to see why most teenagers do not reach their peak bone mass. The effects of being shortchanged on calcium and vitamin D go beyond the risk of osteoporosis in the future. There may be a price to pay much sooner. Recent Mayo Clinic studies report that nearly all of the young people with chronic pain have severe vitamin D deficiency and that, compared with 30 years ago, there has been an alarming rise in children's forearm fractures.

Do all children need supplements? Can they get all the nutrients they need from food? They can if they follow the Fountain of Youth program. If not, they certainly need foods fortified with high levels of D and other nutrients, or they need to take supplements that will provide 2,000 IU per day of D.

In a study that followed thousands of women over a period of 17 years, Drs. Feskanick and Willet showed that those who consumed the most milk and dairy products had the most fractures; so dairy is certainly not the answer. The dairy lobby has failed to publish any long-term studies showing that consuming high levels of dairy products can prevent obesity and fractures. They do a lot of advertising, but there's little convincing data.

Are you getting enough D? Half the people in the U.S. are not getting even 200 IU of D. Virtually all experts agree that this is not nearly enough. That's bad news for your bones, since your body needs this vitamin to process calcium efficiently, said Dr. Robert Heaney, a friend and professor of medicine at Creighton University in Omaha. In 2003, he compared the effects of giving postmenopausal women vitamin D supplements for one year, followed by one year with no supplements. The results were clear — with higher vitamin D blood levels, the women absorbed 65% more calcium.

Dr. Heaney and other experts advocate raising the RDA for vitamin D: "Getting too little has been linked to many chronic disorders, from osteoporosis, to type-I and type- II diabetes, and even cancer, so deficiency is a huge health threat," adding that the best protection for children is 1,800 IU daily.

Unfortunately, this nutrient is found in relatively few foods that people like to eat, said Dr. Heaney. While people can get vitamin D naturally through sun exposure, that's not always possible or even a good idea, especially if you are prone to sunburn. In the northern U.S., outdoor workers like lifeguards or landscape workers get plenty of vitamin D in the summer, but it doesn't last through the winter, when the sun is lower on the horizon. Studies show that skin production of vitamin D dwindles in older people, even if they are sun worshippers; suggesting that a supplement might be the best way to safeguard their bone health. Even people who live in Arizona are often deficient in vitamin D, since they usually avoid exposing their pale skin to the sun. In a later chapter, we will discuss just how much vitamin D is enough.

CHAPTER FOUR

HOW OUR BONES GOT INTO THIS MESS

> *"Many of the physical, emotional, and financial costs of bone disease and fractures can be avoided."*
>
> \- United States Surgeon General

From the start of the Industrial Revolution until about 70 years ago, a large percentage of children in big cities were born with a mysterious disease that caused soft bones and excruciating pain. Often the deformities were so severe that doctors needed to deliver the babies by Caesarean section. The bone problem came to be called "rickets." After many years, doctors found that rickets could be cured or prevented with adequate sunlight or vitamin D. The richest known source of vitamin D was cod liver oil, containing omega-3 fatty acids and retinol vitamin A at rather substantial levels. As time went by, scientists noticed that vitamin D, unlike any other vitamin or mineral, turned into a powerful hormone in the body.

Your skin contains compounds that can be converted into vitamin D when exposed to ultraviolet or full spectrum light. With abundant exposure to noonday sun, you do not need to depend upon foods for vitamin D. However, you need to expose 30% of your skin to 30 minutes of sunlight about three times a week. By doing this, depending on the angle and intensity of the sun, you can generate roughly

19,000 units of D per day. People who are out in the sun every day, much like 18th and 19th Century farmers, never suffer from too much vitamin D. However, fear of developing skin cancer or leathery skin prevents many people from enjoying and benefiting from the noontime sun.

Vitamin D toxicity myth

For years, people have talked about vitamin D toxicity, actually referring to problems from too much cod liver oil. Lots of cod liver oil contains toxic oxidized fatty acids and way too much vitamin A. Too much Vitamin A from animal sources contributes to huge problems for humans, including osteoporosis. However, vitamin A from plants, beta-carotene, doesn't cause problems even at very high doses. It simply gives the skin a yellow tint and if the amount is cut back the skin color clears up.

People have gotten too much vitamin D from injections and also can have problems from using vitamin D2, a synthetic product. We don't recommend using D2, unless it is impossible to get D3. **In this book, when we say vitamin D, we mean D3.**

There's a curious account of two Canadian men ingesting an incredibly large amount of D3 without serious results. Reading like scenes from "Arsenic & Old Lace," a wife of one of the men, who had a job adding vitamin D to milk, one day read on the label that D was extremely toxic. She had tired of living with her husband and father-in-law and decided to do away with them. She brought the pure vitamin D home and "accidentally" put it in the sugar bowl, knowing that the men loved ice tea and added a lot of sugar to it. After seven months the men checked into a hospital complaining of digestive problems and diarrhea. Doctors became suspicious and found extraordinarily high calcium levels in their blood. Further evaluations by Dr. Reinhold Vieth revealed that they also had extremely high vitamin D levels in their blood. Dr. Vieth checked all of their foods for vitamin D and discovered that the men had been consuming 1.7 million units of vitamin D per day for seven months from the sugar bowl. Both men were treated and released from the hospital, and they were fine. So much for toxicity of vitamin D. To get this much vitamin D from highly fortified foods, you would need to spend hundreds of dollars a day and you would have to make a conscious effort to take exorbitant amounts.

Ancestors had few D deficiency problems

Throughout known history, before factory and office jobs, our ancestors lived in abundant sunshine. There was no choice. While gardening, hunting, gathering or visiting a neighboring tribe seeking a suitable mate, they always got a lot of sunshine and usually didn't wear a lot of clothes nor used sun block. Because their diet was devoid of processed, refined foods and they got a lot of exercise, it seems they didn't get much skin cancer, either. Amazing, huh?

In the 1920s, medical scientists noted that one teaspoon of cod liver oil would prevent rickets. The recommended amount of 200-400 units of vitamin D was established as the recommended daily allowance (RDA) for a child or adult, based on the amount found in one teaspoon of cod liver oil. Curiously, they didn't take into account that an adult weighs 25 times as much as a baby. Nor did they know that vitamin

D becomes a super-hormone and controls the activities of every cell in the human body and that deficiency could contribute to diabetes, arthritis, heart disease, and osteoporosis. Even with the thousands of research studies that have been done, we are still saddled with the pseudo-scientific thinking from the 1920s. It's time for a change.

D helps more than just your bones

During the 1990s, many fine researchers stepped forward and published outstanding papers. A few of the leaders are Dr. Heaney, Dr. Vieth, Dr. Holick and Dr. Hollis. They have made us aware that:

1. Vitamin D is more than just a bone nutrient.

2. Historically, people who spend a good deal of time outdoors have been getting more than 10,000 IU per day without any problems.

3. The optimum level of vitamin D is the amount that will maintain a person's blood level of 25 Hydroxy D at 100 to 150 nmol/l. (Higher levels get you closer to the **Fountain of Youth** in my opinion.)

4. It takes more vitamin D than expected to reach this level, probably between 5,000 to 10,000 IU per day. It depends on your metabolism; everyone is different.

5. The potential for toxicity of vitamin D3 has been greatly overstated, whereas the potential toxicity of a dose of vitamin A, from animal sources just 40% above RDA, has been curiously ignored. Could it be because milk has so much animal source vitamin A in it?

6. Winter time production of D is near nonexistent levels unless you live south of Florida and north of Rio de Janeiro.

7. Populations in all parts of the world are lacking in vitamin D. In sunny climates, most women consciously avoid the sun because they want their skin tone to be as light as possible.

8. Milk is a poor vehicle for delivering vitamin D. The FDA found that those who consumed the most milk had no more vitamin D in their blood that those who consumed *no* milk. Evidently, absorption is a problem because of curd formation.

9. Fatty fish is not a good alternative, because most people avoid eating the fat, which is where the vitamin D is found. An exception is good tasting sardines that are very difficult to find.

10. Keep tuned, for new research is being discovered every day. On December 16, 2005 a study was released showing that vitamin D can increase lung capacity by 33%. Amazing! This is extremely important to all people and especially to athletes.

Science of vitamin D is very strong

If you would like to read scientific abstracts on vitamin D go to *www.vitaminDinfo.org* or if you just want to read the results of studies, here are some quotes:

Dr. Holick from Boston University and Dr. Brinkley from the University of Wisconsin Osteoporosis Research Center found that "63% of women being treated for osteoporosis are still severely deficient in vitamin D and 20% have broken a bone recently even though they were already being given drugs for osteoporosis. It's time to change how women are being treated for osteoporosis; they should be given high doses of vitamin D supplements, with or without drugs."

Dr. Moore from the Beverage Institute for Health and Wellness found that "only 4% of the people between the ages of 1-51 met or exceeded the ridiculously low, so called 'adequate intake' of 400 IU of vitamin D."

Dr. Jeannine and co-workers from the Department of Internal Medicine in Amsterdam found that people who have serious vitamin D deficiency took from 7 months to 8 years to find a doctor who could give a proper diagnosis. 95% of the doctors were giving wild guesses that the patients had steroid drug deficiencies of all sorts, orthopedic problems or rheumatic diseases. The poor patients went to 20-40 doctors to find a scientifically correct diagnosis. Treatment given by Dr. Jeannine was about 10,000 IU per day and it took people from 1-3 months to become replete with vitamin D (tissue levels of 80 to 120 nmol/l.) These results warn that it is difficult to find a doctor who can recognize a vitamin D deficiency, and it is difficult to find foods that have enough vitamin D in them to do the job. Ask your doctor if he or she has read any books on vitamin D deficiency and its many benefits.

Dr. Peach found that "Taking a patient history with special attention to change in gait, place of birth, vegetarian diet and whether arms were usually covered outdoors was more effective than biochemical tests in screening patients. The bone pain of hypovitaminosis D (deficiency) is usually dull and poorly localized, often beginning in the lower back and later spreading to the pelvis and hips, upper thighs, upper back and ribs. Characteristically, the pain is felt in the bones rather than in the joints. On questioning, patients often complain of muscle weakness and difficulty in walking." *(Editor's note: Sometimes the diagnosis of Fibromyalgia or Multiple Sclerosis is made.)*

Drs. Mylott, Kemp, Bolton and Greenbaum from the University of Wisconsin reported in 2004 that they were finding "a sickness among the children of America that causes excruciating pain, skeletal deformities, failure to thrive, fractures, seizures, irritability, tiredness and refusal to walk." You could call this a disease, but it is really a condition of being very vitamin D deficient. Years ago, when all children played outside in sunshine and clean air, they never developed rickets, but now it is on the rise again.

Do something about these problems

I believe that if "terrorists" forced American children to live on a vitamin D deficient diet, correcting the problem would receive unlimited funding for a "Manhattan-style research project" or maybe even start WWIII. But ignorance, ineptitude and lack of ethics on the part of the food and medical industries are allowing this to happen in every state in America.

First off, 70 years ago, *researchers on vitamin D set the recommended dietary level of vitamin D 10 times too low. It really should be 4,000 IU per day per person today,* according to leading world Vitamin D researchers.

Secondly, milk is the poorest food to fortify because many people can't absorb vitamin D from milk. As stated before, in July, 2004, the FDA reported that heavy milk drinkers had no more vitamin D in their bodies than people who consume no milk. We need to really push for fortification of all foods that people really love to eat, foods like bread, dark non-dairy chocolate, cookies and peanut butter.

Thirdly, cereal grains are an ideal way to provide vitamin D to people, according to experts from Rockefeller and Rutgers University. Natural Ovens Bakery in Manitowoc, WI, is leading the way by sponsoring research showing that if people get 5,000 IU per day from bread, their blood levels of vitamin D can go from near zero to ideal levels within three months. The people who received this amount of vitamin D showed big increases in muscle and bone strength in just one year. None showed any toxicity or elevated calcium levels in blood or urine.

Fixing our bones and attaining the fountain of youth depends upon obtaining adequate levels of vitamin D in our diet, plus all the other nutrients that the body needs. Without enough D, many of the nutrients from fresh whole vegetables, fruits, grains, legumes, nuts and seeds are wasted. Even filtered water and exercise are both much better utilized with adequate levels of vitamin D3.

CHAPTER FIVE

THE MESSAGE IN PAIN

"Prevalence surveys suggest that 9% to 20% of adults in the United States experience chronic pain. Of these, 89% have some degree of long-term or short-term disability, and nearly all have substantially reduced health-related quality of life. Direct and indirect costs related to chronic pain are estimated at $50 billion annually."

- Gregory Plotnikoff, MD, MTS and Joanna M. Quigley, BA
Prevalence of Severe Hypovataminosis D in Patients with Persistent Nonspecific Musculoskeletal Pain

Every time I see someone in pain, I want to cry out to them, "Don't you know about cayenne pepper and vitamin D?" If your golden years are not so great, then you need to read this chapter. Pain can make you feel old before your time, and chronic pain makes you feel old all the time. Pain is not to be looked at as punishment for something you did, but it can be useful as a signal that some part of your body is not happy--deficient, not getting enough nutrients or oxygen. Masking pain with pain killers will not make it go away. It only serves to partially cover the pain. Finding the real cause of the pain, and doing something about it can eliminate it forever. Growing older doesn't have to mean more pain each year. Eliminate the causes and you can have less and less pain each year. Everything is a lot more fun if you don't hurt.

Pain from an old injury is a cry for vitamin D to finally and properly heal old wounds. Only high levels of natural vitamin D3 can do the job.

Pain is the signal...not the problem

However, here's what happens to most of us. We're busy helping others, taking the kids to soccer practice, cooking, cleaning, etc. and a pain in the leg develops. So you think...I'll take an aspirin to relieve the pain. It's likely you forget, or didn't even realize, that you didn't get much sunshine or vitamin D lately. So you take the aspirin and pain is reduced. But after two hours the pain is in the stomach. Should you take another aspirin? Or did the aspirin cause bleeding in the stomach which is causing you to feel pain? Hard to know, but medical authorities know that 40% of the pain Americans suffer is a side effect from a pain-killer drug they have taken. *(See www.drugs.com for a list of side-effects caused by pain killing drugs.)*

Drug side effects are killers

Side effects from drugs are a serious problem. Some senior citizens are spending years in woo-woo land, hardly knowing where they are. Authorities report that over 100,000 people per year not only have a lot of pain, but actually die from legal drugs taken as prescribed. Be careful and use your intelligence and skepticism...ask your doctor a lot of questions if you don't feel a drug is right for you. The challenge is to know if that pain you are having is from a past injury that has not healed properly or the result of the particular pain-killing drug you're taking or something else.

The Mayo Clinic has a special $15,000, 3-week, pain management seminar for people with chronic pain. The clinic tries to get people off as many pain killing drugs as possible, uses bio-feedback and counseling, and reports that the program can reduce the average person's total pain by 50% in just three weeks.

It has been reported that people in Florida take twice as many drugs as people in Minnesota of the same age and health condition. Yet the people in Florida do not get well as fast as those in Minnesota. Why? Experts say it is because people in Florida are over-medicated! Taking more drugs is not the same as having better health.

Pay attention to side effects

Side effects from drugs are a serious and costly health problem. The government reports that the fourth leading cause of death in America is legal drugs being taken *as prescribed*. Many suffer complications, so be careful. Only you can decide whether a drug is right for you. Get as much information as possible, and ask your doctor a lot of questions if you don't feel right about taking a drug. The challenge is to know whether that pain you are having is from a past injury that has not healed properly or is the result of the particular pain-killing drug you're taking.

Pain among employees is costly

Nearly one in three workers suffers from pain that affects not only their health but also their productivity, according to a new study. Researchers surveyed employees of a major Fortune 500 company and found nearly 30% were in pain beyond the normal everyday aches and pains, like toothaches or muscle sprains.

> *"Lack of vitamin D is killing and injuring more people than all of the wars ever fought in the history of mankind."*
>
> \- Paul A. Stitt, M.S., Biochemist

Lost productivity due to performing at less than 100% on the job (presenteeism) as well as missing work days (absenteeism) amounted to about four days a month for those in pain compared with less than half a day for healthy employees. Researchers say the findings confirm that pain in the workplace is a major cause of lost productivity that merits greater attention by employers. Four common pain conditions--headaches, arthritis, back pain and other musculoskeletal problems--cause productivity losses among 13% of the U.S. workforce at a cost of more than $62 billion per year.

Measuring employee pain

In this study, researchers looked at the burden of pain among more than 1,000 employees of a Fortune 500 company based in the Northeast to determine the extent of the problem and identify possible targets for interventions. Researchers measured pain by asking workers how much bodily pain they experienced in the last four weeks and if they were experiencing pain other than common, everyday aches and pains on the day of the survey.

Results showed that nearly 30% of employees were in pain. Pain among employees was linked to a 45% drop in overall physical health and a 23% drop in mental health. Pain was also linked to substantial declines in productivity. Lost productivity caused by healthy employees missing a day or not performing at 100% at work amounted to just more than a third of a day over the previous four weeks. But for those who were in pain, lost productivity from presenteeism and absenteeism totaled about four days. Employees reporting the highest level of pain were also more likely to report one or more accidents at work in the last year compared with healthy employees.

How employees manage pain

Although employees said they used a variety of means to manage their pain - medication, visiting a doctor and exercise - many rated their current pain treatment approach far short of optimal, leaving much room for improvement. Researchers say the greatest room for improvement in pain management was found among those with musculoskeletal pain conditions, such as arthritis. Results of the study appear in the *Journal of Occupational and Environmental Medicine (July 2005; vol 47: pp 658-670)*.

Research done by Drs. Plotnikoff and Quigley at the University of Minnesota found that 93% of the people with chronic pain had severe vitamin D deficiency. They found this to be true in people of all ages, all races and of all classes. This is a study of major importance in trying to find the real cause of pain.

Dr. Gloth at Johns Hopkins University in Baltimore treated five patients with severe pain triggered by light touch or small movements. He gave them injections of high levels of vitamin D and, within seven days, their pain was resolved. Dr. Mascarenhas from Loyola University near Chicago reported that vitamin D deficiency is a major

> *"Nearly one in three workers suffers from pain that affects not only their health but their productivity."*
>
> - Allen, H.
> Journal of Occupational and Environmental Medicine

health issue and said people with persistent, non-specific pain should be given adequate doses of the vitamin for that pain.

Dr. Lewis from London urges all people with chronic lower back pain to be treated with vitamin D, since if left untreated; these patients could require spinal fusion surgery and risk even more surgeries and possible death. He suggests testing all such patients for low vitamin D levels in the blood and correcting the deficiency.

Dr. Holick says that fibromyalgia is just another word for vitamin D deficiency. Same for MS. We have found that if people with these diseases avoid all junk foods and everything from a cow and take 5,000 to 10,000 IU per day of vitamin D, many of their symptoms will be resolved in two months.

Medical researchers found that most doctors do not even look for vitamin D deficiency and that patients spent from 7 months to 8 years before they could find a doctor that diagnosed them properly. Researchers in Switzerland found they had to give patients about 10,000 IU of vitamin D daily for 1-3 months to resolve chronic pain problems.

Here's a success story: Jim had been in pain for many years from an old football injury. He started taking dark chocolate clusters infused with 2,000 IU of D per piece daily. He loved the taste and kept taking it for two months, without noticing any big changes. Then one day, he woke up and the pain was completely gone. It hasn't returned since.

Magic of cayenne pepper

The safest, most effective pain killer I have ever used is plain old cayenne pepper capsules, available in any natural food store. After I had hernia surgery, I took two cayenne pepper capsules every two hours for relieving pain until I didn't need them anymore. Around midnight the day after surgery, the pain got very bad and so I took an Aleve™, but other than that, I had a rapid recovery and was able to walk five miles, albeit slowly, on the third day after surgery. On the fourth day I was able to get through an airport, fly home and I drove my car home from the airport – a trip of two hours. My doctor said he had never seen anyone heal so fast. After two days, he removed the stitches. The doctor thought I had a miraculous recovery, but I told him that rapid healing was a result of good nutrition, cayenne pepper capsules and proper exercise, not magic.

Motion is the best lotion

Moderate exercise is very important. *Motion is the best lotion.* You have to promote good circulation by exercising up to your ability. This means getting the blood flowing to all parts of your body, feeding every organ with nutrients and oxygen they need. Stretching is also very important. Whether you call it yoga or stretching, it helps the body to stay loose. It's wise to set up a routine so you have time to exercise and stretch every day. Adding a little time for meditation, yoga, chi gong or tai chi every day is good for the body, mind and soul.

Treat pain as if it is a signal of a deeper problem – lack of circulation, lack of oxygen or a lack of nutrients, not as a sign that you need to take another pain killer. Remember the Vioxx™ warning and cover-up. You'll be glad if you can find some natural way to prevent the pain in the first place.

Start taking cayenne pepper, massage the affected area, and check with a chiropractor or licensed massage therapist. Take safer pain killers like Aleve™, aspirin or Tylenol™ *for short periods of time* (*never* more than 10 days) at the lowest possible dose (always start with one). Always use caution when dealing with pain killers, none of them is innately safe. *For more detailed scientific information on this subject, go to www.vitaminDinfo.org*

AN ACTUAL CUSTOMER LETTER, DATED SEPTEMBER 22, 2005

Mr. Paul Stitt
Executive Director
Nutritional Resource Foundation
Manitowoc, WI 54220

Dear Mr. Stitt:

I would like to tell you my story about the pain I've experienced in my life. When I was about 14 years old, while working in a hay elevator, I got my legs caught. As I was hung over the edge of the elevator, my face buried in the hay, I felt searing pain, and was afraid that I was going to lose my left leg. The farmer I was working with freed my right leg, and I was sent to the hospital. Both of my legs had been severely pinched at the knees.

Since that time, I have had severe knee pain. I would often swing my feet back and forth to relieve the stiffness, but this provided only temporary relief.

Now, 40 years later, I have learned about the benefits of vitamin D, and how it can help to relieve chronic pain. I eat healthier foods, I walk more and I drink more water. My mobility has improved, and I am virtually pain free.

Thank you for your interest and research into vitamin D and its benefits, and for your concern for the health and well-being of people everywhere.

Sincerely,
Sharon

CHAPTER SIX

VITAMIN D HELPS PREVENT AND TREAT DIABETES

"There is tantalizing evidence that vitamin D may help to prevent childhood diabetes."

- Oliver Gillie, PhD
Medical Researcher

Diabetes seems to be the beginning of most chronic diseases. After developing diabetes, many people develop obesity, then heart disease and arthritis and end up taking a dozen drugs with many aggravating side-effects, but don't eliminate any of their problems. They end up in "treatment" for the rest of their lives with continued pain and suffering. Find a natural means, like changing eating and exercise habits, and avoid all these problems. Studying the book, *Food and Behavior* by Barbara Stitt, can really help you.

Diabetes is a strange disease that comes in two forms: type-I, where the body does not produce any insulin, and type-II, where the body produces a lot of insulin, but responds poorly to it. It's like stepping on the brake in your car and nothing happens. Insulin regulates the glucose supply in your body for the cells that burn this special sugar for energy. If the sugar supply is not regulated, you have either too much glucose (like our brakeless car) or not enough (car won't go).

It's important to prevent diabetes

It is extremely important to prevent diabetes in every child. Diabetes is often the forerunner to erratic behavior and obesity in children, which can lead to a lifetime of bad self-image, taunting from other children and other humongous problems.

One cause of type-I diabetes

For years researchers have been mystified by the causes of diabetes. Recent research in Finland, which has the highest reported incidence of type-I in the world, has given us clues. Northern Finland receives only two hours of sunlight daily during the winter. A Finnish study of 12,000 babies born in 1966 found those who were given the recommended amounts of vitamin D supplement (2,000 IU at that time) had an 88% reduced risk of developing diabetes.

Researchers, following these children for over 30 years, found that only 81 out of the 12,000 had been diagnosed with diabetes during the study. Children were monitored for vitamin D intake in the first year, and classed as below, within or above the recommended amount. It was found that children who took any amount of vitamin D had a significantly lower rate of diabetes than those who did not.

Children who were given supplements regularly reduced their risk by 80%. Those with rickets in the first year of life (linked to vitamin D deficiency) had a three-fold risk of developing diabetes. This is the first large-scale study to follow children's diet and their later development of diabetes.

We don't know what causes the destruction of insulin secreting cells in the pancreas and the development of type-I diabetes. Type-I diabetes is an autoimmune disease, where the immune system destroys its own cells. However, we do know that vitamin D is an immune suppressing agent and may help prevent an overly aggressive response from the immune system.

Contributory causes of diabetes

Type-II or adult onset diabetes has several contributory causes, including the consumption of high glycemic index foods that turn into glucose too fast in your body. Eating them is like putting racing fuel in your car; your car goes so fast that it burns itself out. The other main cause is eating foods that have few nutrients and very little fiber, *such as fast foods*. If your body has no nutrients to build new cells it just turns on itself and starts tearing it down. Lack of fiber in the diet also causes problems in the digestive process. If you have diabetes, you're more at risk for osteoporosis, bone fractures and many other painful illnesses.

My friend, Dr. Richard Anderson with the USDA, found that 900 mcg of chromium a day can eliminate many of the symptoms of diabetes. He also found that half a teaspoon a day of cinnamon can help people with diabetes. He's a good scientist, worth listening to.

Diabetes weakens the bones

In the May 2005 *American Journal of Clinical Nutrition*, Ken C. Chiu and his colleagues from the University of California, Los Angeles, reported that the lower the vitamin

D, the greater the risk of type-I diabetes. Chiu's team found that increasing a person's blood concentration of vitamin D from 25 nmol/l to about 75 nmol/l (increase diet level from 400 IU to 2,000 IU) would "improve insulin sensitivity by 60%," a greater increase than many anti-diabetes drugs provide. Increasing the intake to 4,000-5,000 IU daily could significantly improve these results.

Nicodemus at the University of Minnesota found that women with type-I diabetes were 12 times more likely to experience a hip fracture than women who don't have diabetes. Those with type-II have double the risk.

In Norway, Dr. Forsen found that women with type-I diabetes were seven times more likely to break a hip. Older women with type-II diabetes were 150% more likely to break a leg, whether they took their medicine or not. Dr. Schwartz's group in California found about the same results: those on insulin had many more foot fractures. The lesson here is to *avoid the type of diet that brings on diabetes.*

Vitamin D helps prevent diabetes

Dr. Pozzilli of Mexico found that lack of vitamin D was a cause of diabetes and that children born with type-I diabetes should be treated with vitamin D.

Dr. Grant from the Sunlight Nutrition and Health Research Center in San Francisco reports there's strong evidence of the *protective effect of vitamin D against* several bone diseases, muscle weakness, more than a dozen types of internal cancers, multiple sclerosis, and type-I diabetes mellitus.

Dr. Mathieu from Belgium found lack of vitamin D leads to type-I and type-II diabetes and to a lowered production of insulin where the blood sugar level cannot be controlled.

Dr. de Souza-Santos from Brazil found that vitamin D reduced the high blood sugar level to normal levels.

Dr. Peterrlik from the University of Medicine, Vienna, Austria, found that "vitamin D deficits increase the risk of cancer, particularly of colon, breast and prostate gland, of chronic inflammatory and autoimmune diseases (e.g. insulin-dependent diabetes mellitus, inflammatory bowel disease, multiple sclerosis), as well as of metabolic disorders (metabolic syndrome, hypertension). That's a whole lot of problems.

Dr. Harris from the New England Research Institute found that 400 IU per day of D did *not* prevent diabetes, but that 2,000 IU per day *did*.

Cayenne is good for people with poor circulation from diabetes

Several years ago, a woman came to us seeking information. Her diabetes had killed the blood circulation in her feet to the point where one foot was amputated the previous year. She asked if we could help her so she wouldn't lose her other foot. I told her about our great success with cayenne pepper in improving circulation. She took one capsule and could feel the improved circulation within 15 minutes. She took 3 capsules a day, and in 5 weeks, her circulation was greatly improved. Her leg was no longer black and blue and was warm as toast. She was a delighted woman as the surgery was cancelled and she still has her foot. Sometimes, it is the simplest things that can help people.

Cow's milk worsens diabetes

A Dr. Borissova gave 2,000 IU of vitamin D to people with type-II diabetes. After just one month, insulin levels improved 34% and insulin responsiveness was increased. Dr. Virtanen from Finland found that *cow's milk produced an antibody that destroyed the part of the body that produces insulin*. He found that cow's milk products dramatically increased the risk of diabetes.

Control blood sugar to avoid heart attacks, strokes

Dr. David M. Nathan of Harvard Medical School says that diabetics who tightly control their blood sugar levels can cut their risk of heart attacks and strokes in half. A long-awaited, federally-funded study, that shows nearly 1,400 diabetics who have been followed for more than a decade, provides the first direct evidence that the risk of the most serious complications of the disease, affecting millions of Americans, can be minimized by aggressive treatment.

"This is the most important diabetes news of the year," said Dr. Nathan, who co-chaired the study, published in the January, 2006, issue of the *New England Journal of Medicine*. "This is the remaining piece of the puzzle with regard to our ability to take the teeth out of diabetes and make it a less dangerous disease." Nearly 21 million Americans have diabetes, and the number is rising because of the increasing number of elderly and obese people.

To strictly control blood sugar, lifestyle improvements are much more effective than an insulin pump, said my niece who works for a medical doctor who fits people with insulin pumps. Diabetics need to put themselves on a healthy diet of high levels of vitamin D, high in fiber and natural foods, and avoid all dairy products, and foods made with bleached white flour, hydrogenated fats and corn syrup. A little natural sugar like crystalline fructose, sucrose, and real maple syrup are fine in small amounts as long as the total diet is very high in all essential nutrients. When your future life is at stake, it's worth making radical changes like this. For help, check out the *Natural Ovens Cookbook* and Barbara Stitt's, *Food and Behavior*, available by calling 800-772-0730.

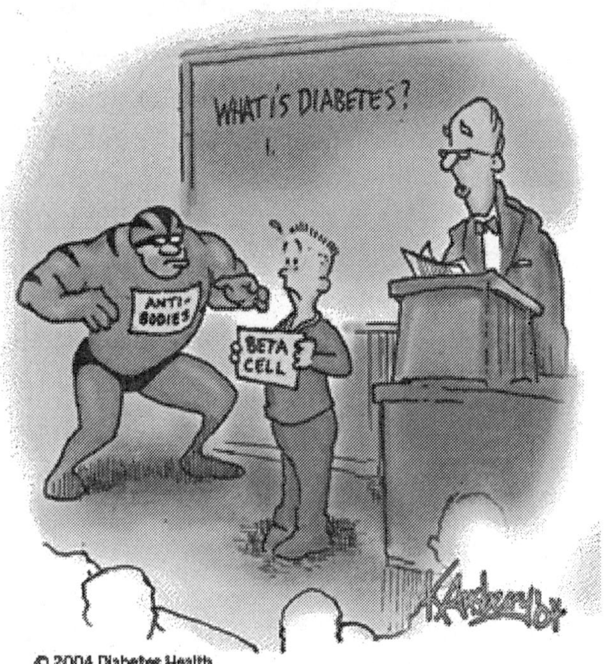

"...and to demonstrate the immune system's devastating attack on the body's insulin-producing beta cells, we will now recreate this encounter with the help of Milton Pitts and Bruno the Mangler."

Diabetes Health. Printed with permission.

CHAPTER SEVEN

D DEFICIENCY IN PEOPLE OF COLOR AN EPIDEMIC

> "*African American men and women have greater prevalence of vitamin D insufficiency, which may be a factor in their susceptibility to certain cancers. New recommendations for Vitamin D should be made for the otherwise healthy populations in greatest need of dietary Vitamin D due to lack of adequate sun exposure.*
>
> Calvo, MS and Whiting, SJ,
> College of Pharmacy and Nutrition,
> University of Saskatchewan, Saskatoon, Saskatchewan, Canada

Vitamin D deficiency in people of color has reached epidemic proportions. It has nothing to do with race, but rather skin pigmentation, nature's way to protect those who normally reside in sunny, tropical climates. The darker the skin, the more exposure from the sun it needs to make vitamin D.

Dr. Oz told Oprah on her show that she had a natural sun block of 500. Dr. Holick recently said that African-Americans absorb only 2%-50% as much of the UV from the sun as those with lighter skin. People with darker skin are generally more deficient in vitamin D than Caucasians and experience twice as much chronic pain, bone fractures, prostate, ovarian and breast cancer, heart disease, diabetes and many other chronic maladies. Dark-skinned people living in sunny places like Jamaica and Nigeria are often deficient in vitamin D, and those living in northern climates are much worse off. Researchers believe darker-skinned people need more D than light-skinned people. The recommended level set by the government is *far too low* to prevent vitamin D deficiency even for those with lighter skin. Women of color need about 5,000 IU per day, not the 100-200 most get.

Dark skinned people don't necessarily have more fractures than pale skins, but they have twice as many of the other problems associated with vitamin D deficiency – arthritis, breast, uterine, colon and prostate cancer, diabetes, arthritis, etc.

> "*Being deprived of vitamin D is like being deprived of Life, Liberty, and the Pursuit of Happiness* "
>
> - Paul A Stitt, M.S., Biochemist

Immigrants in real danger

Immigrant women who practice orthodox religions by keeping their bodies and faces completely covered have severe vitamin D deficiency. When I see a woman fully covered, I want to tell her about the benefits of vitamin D, but I know it would be improper for me to approach her. Please help by sharing what you have learned with any of these women.

How big is the problem?

Thank God for Bruce Hollis, who has been doing feeding studies on people of color. And for John Cannell, M.D., who is suing the FDA for genocide against all people of color by not warning them of the health dangers of vitamin D deficiency by setting the "adequate intake" level criminally low.

Dr. Hollis found that 2,000 IU of D daily was not nearly enough for lactating women of color, but that 4,000 IU per day would raise their serum to the adequate range. This can help prevent soft, painful bones in the baby, help prevent diabetes, and improve learning ability in the child. Dr. Hollis urges the government to raise the recommended level so it's at least adequate to prevent chronic diseases. He found 10,000 IU per day for five months in women of color was adequate and did not raise serum levels too high.

Dr. Aloia of Chicago fed African-American post-menopausal women 2,000 IU per day of vitamin D, plus 1,500 mg/day of calcium for two years. He found no increases in bone mineral density for two reasons: 2,000 IU of D per day is not enough for people who have been deficient in D for 50 years, and 1,500 mg/day is too much calcium. Excess calcium blocks vitamin D from being activated in the body. Many doctors who are partially educated in this field make this same mistake; thinking that more calcium is always better. It becomes toxic at high levels and blocks absorption of iron, zinc, magnesium, etc. Veterinarians use high levels of ionized calcium to euthanize cats.

Dr. S. Harris from Tufts University thinks the government should do more to educate people of color as well as whites on the benefits of adequate vitamin D. Dr. Faraj found that 83% of the people who came to a pain clinic in Saudi Arabia were deficient in vitamin D. Patients' pain was reduced or completely eliminated when they were given adequate vitamin D. Dr. Abdullah found that 83% of the teenagers in Saudi Arabia, a rich and sunny country, had vitamin D deficiency because they covered up with clothing.

Dr. Holvik from Oslo conducted a study on immigrant groups living in Sweden and found that "there is widespread vitamin D deficiency in both men and women born in Turkey, Sri Lanka, Iran, Pakistan and Vietnam residing in Oslo." Their average serum level was 29, only 1/4th of what is needed; it should be 100 nmol/l. Those that were most obese had the lowest level of vitamin D.

Dr. Nesby-O'Dell from Center for Disease Control and Prevention in Atlanta reported that 42% of dark skinned people are extremely deficient in vitamin D and about 95% have a serum level below 100nmol/l; a level necessary to prevent osteoporosis, chronic pain, diabetes and autoimmune diseases.

For more detailed scientific information on this subject, go www.vitaminDinfo.org

CHAPTER 8

FDA MORE ENLIGHTENED ABOUT VITAMIN D SUPPLEMENT

> "*If sunlight were really bad for us, we'd be nocturnal creatures like mice.*"
>
> - Francis Gasparro,
> professor of dermatology,
> Thomas Jefferson University

The FDA has a reputation of opposing all uses of vitamin supplements. The people at FDA *compliance* have worked hard to shut down medical doctors that prescribe supplements and alternative treatments for most diseases, regardless of how strong the supporting scientific evidence. However, *the internal* FDA research experts on vitamin D are some of the highest caliber and most forward thinking individuals that I have ever met. Specifically, Dr. Mona Calvo and her associates have been working tirelessly to get the FDA's advisory board to wake up and promote more vitamin D consumption by all Americans.

In 2005, the FDA reported that globally, there is a high prevalence of vitamin D insufficiency, a re-emergence of rickets, and growing scientific evidence that links low circulating vitamin D to increased risk of osteoporosis, diabetes, cancer and autoimmune disorders. Dr. Calvo and colleagues have been working for years to raise the recommended intake for vitamin D. Here are some quotes from FDA published work:

J Steroid Biochem Mol Biol. 2005 Oct; 97(1-2):7-12

High prevalence of vitamin D insufficiency and the re-emergence of rickets have been observed worldwide. For many countries without mandatory staple food fortification, Vitamin D intake is often too low to sustain healthy circulating levels of vitamin D. Supplement use can significantly increase vitamin D intakes across all age and gender groups. African-American men and women have greater prevalence of vitamin D insufficiency, which *may* be a factor in their susceptibility to certain cancers. New recommendations for vitamin D should be made for the otherwise healthy populations in greatest need of dietary vitamin D due to lack of adequate sun exposure.

J Nutr. 2005 Feb;135(2):310-6.

Global high prevalence of vitamin D insufficiency and re-emergence of rickets and the growing scientific evidence links low circulating vitamin D to increased risk of osteoporosis, diabetes, cancer and autoimmune disorders. Concern over increased risk of melanoma with unprotected UVB exposure has led to the alternative recommendation that sufficient vitamin D should be supplied through dietary sources alone. It is evident from our review that vitamin D intake is often way too low to sustain healthy circulating levels of vitamin D in countries without mandatory staple food fortification.

Even in countries that do fortify foods, vitamin D intakes are low in some groups due to their unique dietary patterns, such as a vegetarian diet which would eliminate egg yolks and fish such as sardines, limit use of dietary supplements, or loss of *traditional* high fish intakes. Recent studies demonstrate safety and efficacy of community-based vitamin D supplementation trials and food staple. Reliance on the world food supply as an alternative to UVB exposure will necessitate greater availability of fortified food staples, dietary supplement use, and/or change in dietary patterns to consume more fatty fish.

> *"The importance of beginning prevention at a very young age and continuing throughout life is now well understood."*
>
> \- United States Surgeon General

J Nutr. 2005 Feb;135(2):304-9.

1997 determination of vitamin D requirements and status was more conjecture than science. The circulating metabolite vitamin D is the major static indicator of vitamin D status. Using its response to diet in the absence of sun exposure, a dose-response study suggests a mean requirement of at least 500 IU (12.5 microg) from which an RDA could be set.

PS: This means at an intake of 500 IU daily, only 50% of the population will have minimum serum vitamin D levels. The law says that recommended dietary intake level must meet the needs of virtually all people.

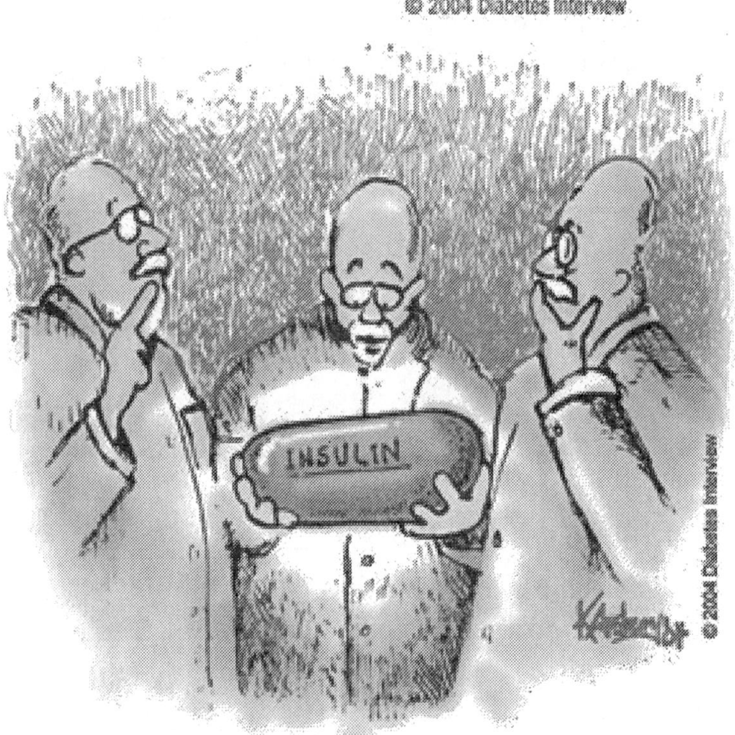

Despite the valiant efforts of the research group, the insulin suppository still had one major drawback.

Diabetes Health. Printed with permission.

Bone. 2002 May;30(5):771-7.

Data from 18,875 individuals examined in the Third National Health and Nutrition Examination Survey (NHANES III 1988-1994) was used to assess the vitamin D status of selected groups of the free living U.S. adolescent and adult population.

Up to 57% of this population had *below* the minimum adequate level. Vitamin D insufficiency is common in these populations. Of particular interest is that insufficiency occurred fairly frequently in younger individuals, especially in the winter and lower latitude population.

This data shows a terrible indictment of the present vitamin D situation in America, but you really can't fault the FDA people at the Center for Food Safety and Applied Nutrition.

CHAPTER NINE

PROTECT YOURSELF FROM OSTEOPOROSIS

"Everyone should know that vitamin D is critical to the formation and maintenance of normal bones. Even if people consume enough calcium, they cannot build and maintain bone mass if they are deficient in vitamin D."

- Jane E. Brody
New York Times health writer

Nearly everyone's greatest fear is to end up with a hunched back and fragile bones. It's a 21st Century disease that's growing by leaps and bounds. It's truly a lifestyle disease, brought on by a combination of factors, not just a single cause. The largest factor is the lack of sunshine exposure on our skin, and a noticeable lack of vitamin D in nearly all our foods. Government inertia is making the problem even worse, and the Institute of Medicine's failure to recognize that the recommended intake of vitamin D, set 70 years ago, was 5-10 times too low to meet the needs of people who get little sun exposure.

Every time I see someone hunched over with osteoporosis, I want to rush over and say: "Wake up, you need lots of vitamin D." Their likely response, "but my doctor says..." I would ask, "Has your doctor studied nutrition?" Sometimes I will win them over, but so many have such blind trust in the medical and drug establishment that they don't listen. I hope the debacle about Merck falsifying reports will make people wake up and seek other means to become pain free without resorting to more and more drugs.

Osteoporosis is the symbol of growing old in many people's minds. Many women think it's inevitable, especially if their mother had it. It is the worst of all fates: imagine yourself lonely, without friends or companion, full of pain and the fear that you might fall, break a bone, never heal and have unending pain for the rest of your natural life. Not a pretty picture. From what we know today, it can be avoided or even reversed with forethought and planning based on sound information.

Garbage-in, garbage-out

The healthfulness of the American diet has taken a plunge in the last 50 years. Fast food companies and associates have led us down a slippery slope. They've conditioned the American consumer to believe that foods good for them must taste bad. Without any objection from the medical profession, they want us to believe that what we eat has little to do with our health today or in the future. We wouldn't feed food to our pets that is void of nutrition, yet that's a lot of what we feed ourselves. Remember the old saying about computers — garbage-in, garbage-out? Everything we eat affects our body, mind and spirit, today and in the future.

Some medical experts say, "We don't really know what causes osteoporosis." In a sense that's true because it sneaks up on us over a period of 20-40 years. Yet, if you know what to look for, the signs are there. You inherited genes from your mother. Did she have osteoporosis? A better question would be: do you eat the same kinds of foods as your mother did, or is your diet better or worse?

Take this helpful quiz

1. Do you have chronic pain every week?
2. Do you use any type of pain killer on a weekly or daily basis?
3. Did your mother lose height as she aged?
4. Are your muscles weaker now than they were 10 years ago?
5. Have you suffered a fracture?
6. Do you suffer from PMS?
7. Have you had your blood checked for 25 Hydroxy D level?

If you answered yes to any of the first 6 questions, then you should follow with question 7 action.

What about bone density?

We didn't include a question about bone density; I have not found it to be a very reliable test. People with high density bones often have broken bones. Others, like my wife, have a very low bone density according to one test, yet she has survived five serious falls in the last 25 years without breaking a single bone. Most women would have had multiple fractures, long stays in the hospital and excruciating pain. How did Barbara avoid bone fractures and breaks? She practices a healthy lifestyle; we avoid processed and refined foods and all dairy products. We eat foods highly fortified with vitamin D, including dark chocolates, and exercise daily together.

Vitamin D can turn fat into bone

Gina Kolata wrote a most interesting article about osteoporosis, published in the July, 2005, *New York Times.* She reported that three different U.S. laboratories found that, as people age with osteoporosis, their bones fill with fat. In fact they get so packed with fat they can burst with the smallest bump. However, if you take the marrow fat out of the bone and add vitamin D to it, you can actually see bone cells start to form from the fat. Researchers also reported that if people consumed adequate D throughout their lives, the inner part of their bones would not fill with fat. Want to keep fat out of your bones? Want to turn your fat into bone? Just take enough D and/or spend 15 minutes on each side in high sun (10am-2pm) in a bikini.

What's the real cause of osteoporosis?

These scientists have provided clues about osteoporosis:

Dr. Holick from Boston University found vitamin D reduces body sway and bone fractures in the elderly.

Dr. Harrington at the University of Wisconsin found that most people who have hip fractures are not being tested for osteoporosis and those that were tested were not given vitamin D.

Dr. Turkoski reported that women should follow a good diet that includes vitamin D, egg yolks, sardines, and dark chocolates with added vitamin D, and do weight-bearing exercise. Estrogen therapy is not recommended for treating osteoporosis.

Dr. Keizak reported that men often have osteoporosis, but are much less often diagnosed or treated for the disease.

> *"Physical activity and adequate calcium and vitamin D intake are known to be major contributors to bone health for individuals of all ages."*
>
> - United States Surgeon General

Dr. Mary Elliot from the University of Wisconsin says that osteoporosis treatment involves improving the overall diet, exercising and taking vitamin D and some calcium.

Dr. Munger reported that not having enough protein in the diet increased the risk of hip fractures by 69% in a study of 102,000 postmenopausal women. *Excess protein* can also *increase the risk* for osteoporosis. 45-50 grams of protein per day is about the right amount.

Dr. Simon from Brigham and Women's Hospital in Boston reports that "correction of vitamin D deficiency is an inexpensive task and may require education of clinicians as well as the public. In sum, vitamin D deficiency is prevalent in the elderly and, to correct the adverse skeletal effects, it should be diagnosed, treated and prevented."

Dr. Pfeifer from Germany reported that people who have trouble getting out of a chair or climbing steps need more vitamin D, and possibly more calcium and magnesium.

Dr. Gennari from University of Sienna in Italy reports that people at risk need at least 800 IU of D and a total of 700 mg. calcium per day. To overcome a long-standing deficiency of D, 5,000 IU per day for three months would work.

In the year 2005 alone, 28 peer-reviewed scientific articles were published on the lack of vitamin D in the diet and the increased risk of osteoporosis. Here's a sampling of the results:

Dr. Holick from Boston University and Dr. Binkley, University of Wisconsin's Osteoporosis Clinical Research program, concluded that "the prevalence of vitamin D inadequacy in postmenopausal women in North America, who are receiving medication to forestall or treat osteoporosis, is unacceptably high. Both physicians and the public need to be better educated about how to optimize vitamin D supplementation in these women." That is pretty blunt; it seems that doctors and patients have not gotten the message yet.

Drs. Shaker and Lukert from St. Lukes Medical Center in Milwaukee report that excess steroids can cause osteoporosis and fractures. Even low doses of oral glucocorticoids may be associated with bone loss. Patients should be treated with adequate calcium, magnesium, and vitamin D.

Dr. Simoleei and associates from HealthEast Osteoporosis Care, Woodbury, MN, found a very high percentage of people who break a bone from a minor fall have very low levels of vitamin D in their systems.

Dr. Vieth, long-time researcher of vitamin D, says that osteoporosis can be largely prevented by increasing physical activity, improving nutritional intake, and increasing vitamin D intake to at least 1,000 IU per day. (Personally, he told me that he takes 8,000 IU per day.)

Dr. Munns of Children's Hospital in Sydney, Australia, says that chronically ill children most often have osteoporosis that can be corrected by giving adequate vitamin D, calcium, magnesium and other nutrients.

Dr. Hirota from Japan reports the nutritional condition of the patient affects how well the drugs will work.

Dr. Zochling from the Institute of Bone and Joint Research, University of Sydney, Australia, reports that many people in nursing homes who receive adequate overall nutrition are still vitamin D deficient.

Dr. Bulut from Turkey found that people with MS have very low levels of vitamin D.

Dr. Bertone-Johnson of the Department of Public Health in Amherst, MA, found that low levels of vitamin D dramatically increased the risk of premenstrual syndrome. Since D also reduces the risk of osteoporosis, she suggested that young women increase their D intake.

Dr. Moyad from the University of Michigan Medical Center found that omega-3 fatty acids, as found in flax and fish, reduced the risk of osteoporosis and other diseases.

Dr. Nieves of the Regional Bone Center in New York reported that the micronutrient needs for optimizing bone health can be easily met by a healthy diet high in fruits and vegetables to ensure adequate intakes for magnesium, potassium, vitamin C, vitamin K and other potentially important nutrients. Healthcare professionals need to be aware of the importance of adequate calcium and vitamin D intakes (easily monitored by serum 25(OH)D) for optimal bone health, as well as the prevention of falls and fractures).

Dr. Peterlik from the University of Medicine in Vienna, Austria, reported that lack of vitamin D and calcium may lead to many different chronic diseases, not just osteoporosis.

Dr. Montero-Odasso of the Geriatric Medicine Program, Hospital Italiano de Buenos Aires, Argentina, observed: "We expect that this new information about the importance of vitamin D in the elderly will stimulate an innovative approach to the problem of falls and fractures which will constitute a significant reduction of the burden to public health budgets worldwide."

I think you get the idea. Treating the real cause of osteoporos — vitamin D deficiency — will improve the health of all people worldwide. This idea has very strong scientific backing. For more detailed scientific information on this subject, go to *www.vitaminDinfo.org*

CHAPTER 10

BUILD MUSCLES WITHOUT EXTRA EXERCISING

"Few individuals follow the recommendation for physical activity, vitamin D, calcium, vitamins and other nutrients needed to maintain healthy bones."

- United States Surgeon General

I had always believed that you couldn't build muscle strength without exercising, until my wife proved me wrong. We were planting trees last spring, pulling out dead ones, and driving steel posts to stake the live, leaning ones, when I said to her: "Do you realize that you are carrying twice as many steel posts this year as you could carry last year?" She replied, "I notice that I am much stronger this spring than last spring." She hadn't been doing any extra exercising or weight lifting, but, for about six months, Barbara had been sampling my vitamin D dark chocolates. (I had been experimenting to see how much vitamin D I could add to chocolate without messing up the taste and texture. I made a lot of batches, and, of course, we had to sample all of them.) We believe her extra strength was a direct result of the vitamin D she had been sampling.

Become stronger without stressful exercising

I have had a similar experience. My wife and I have been regular everyday walkers since we got married over 20 years ago. We believe in exercising up to our abilities without overdoing it and causing pain. But this last spring, I couldn't just walk with my wife anymore — I had to do wind sprints. Walking wasn't tough enough for me. For the first time in my life, I really love to do wind sprints, even though I was born in 1940. These personal experiences have convinced me that vitamin D really does help build muscle strength and is the Fountain of Youth. For those who need scientific information to become convinced, I've included some reports below.

If you are D deficient, you may have rather weak muscles, so don't expect to go outside and immediately do a lot of exercising. You have to first build up the level of vitamin D in your blood and muscles. You'll find that your body really wants to exercise. Begin by walking — building up the distance that you walk each week until you are walking at least two miles a day. Your body needs to move to stay healthy. The D helps put you in the mood to move.

Move faster with D

Muscle weakness is a common symptom of severe vitamin D deficiency. Five years ago, nutritional epidemiologist Heike A. Bischoff-Ferrari from Harvard wondered if vitamin D affects muscle function in apparently healthy people as well. So, she measured vitamin D blood concentrations in elderly men and women and found that individuals who had higher readings also had greater muscle strength, could walk faster and get up out of a chair faster.

> *"Vitamin D is a potent force in regulating cell growth, immunity, and energy metabolism."*
>
> - David Feldman
> Stanford University School of Medicine

Bischoff-Ferrari and a team at the University of Basel in Switzerland launched an intervention trial with 122 women in their mid-80s. The researchers administered 800 IU of vitamin D per day to half of them. At the end of three months, each woman was tested for leg strength and rated on how easily she could get up from a chair, walk around an object and sit back down. The group of women who got the vitamin D performed dramatically better on the strength tests, and they had only half as many falls during the trial, according to the researcher report in the February, 2003, *Journal of Bone and Mineral Research*. Falls were reduced by 49% in three months just by adding D to their diet.

More recently, Bischoff-Ferrari combed through a national diet and health survey of some 4,100 men and women aged 60 years and older. The researchers reported in the *American Journal of Clinical Nutrition* that blood concentration of vitamin D directly correlated with leg strength and muscle function in people.

Feel stronger with D

Dr. Visser from the Institute for Research in Extramural Medicine in Germany found that women over age 65 with the most vitamin D in their blood had 257% more muscle strength than others with the least D.

Dr. Stahelin from Switzerland found that senior citizens with the most D had 49% fewer falls in a nursing home. The people with the weakest muscles and most falls before the experiment benefited the most.

Dr. Verhaar from the Netherlands found that vitamin D deficiency leads to a loss of muscle fibers and shrinking of muscles. Giving vitamin D leads to improved muscle strength and increased walking distance.

Dr. Mowe, Aker University Hospital in Oslo, Norway, found that the lack of vitamin D in muscles lead to decreased muscle strength, and increased disability in nursing home residents. Disability levels decreased when adequate D was added to the diet.

Dr. Meyer from the National Health Screening Service in Oslo, Norway, reported that Oslo has the highest incidence of hip fractures in the world. He found it was related to extra skinny people who smoked, ate fewer meals per day and had reduced intake of Vitamin D. *(I guess this is a warning not to try to look like a Norwegian model.)*

Weight lifter success story

A weight lifter friend of mine told me that secretly he has been using high levels of vitamin D to legally build up his muscle strength. He found that it really works, but he doesn't want his opponents to know what he is doing. I am not the least bit surprised that it really works for him. The nice thing is that there are virtually no harmful side effects if it is consumed on a regular basis in food. A few problems have arisen when people took high dose injections with vitamin D2--*the synthetic version.* D3 is the one and only version we recommend.

"Exercise not only helps me to lower my blood-
glucose levels... it also helps me to meet
cute guys like you."
© 2004 Diabetes Health

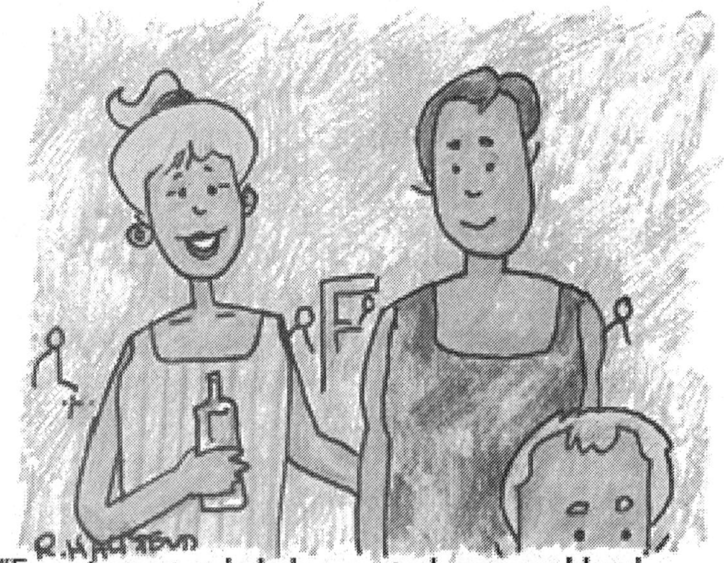

Diabetes Health. Reprinted with permission.

CHAPTER ELEVEN

ARTHRITIS DOESN'T HAVE TO BE THE PRICE OF AGING

"Less than 25% of the people that have a hip fracture were given advice about calcium and vitamin D. Most physicians do not even discuss osteoporosis with a patient after a hip fracture."

- United States Surgeon General

Many consider arthritis to be the price of growing old. A disease on the rise, some folks wear it like a badge and proudly exclaim: "I've had both knees replaced by the best surgeon in the whole world." One wonders where all of the second best surgeons live and work. I'm sure it is not in my hometown.

According to recent data gathered by the Center for Disease Control and Prevention, arthritis is the leading cause of disability in the United States. Arthritis affects about 40% of Americans and 50% of people worldwide. This ailment is more common than cancer or heart disease, and it dates back thousands of years. It is believed that the famous Roman baths were created not only for hygiene purposes, but to help people ease the aches and pains in their joints.

Every time I see someone limping and in pain, I want to ask them if they're getting enough vitamin D to help heal their old injuries and stop the pain. I met a woman who has had four hip replacements because her hips would not bond. The doctor never once checked to see if she had enough D in her system to heal and bond the new hip to the old bone. Such acts of neglect are criminal. Don't just trust your doctor to know the truth about how vitamin D can help you heal and get out of pain. You've got to take charge of your own health.

What is arthritis and how do you get it?

There are two most common forms of arthritis: Rheumatoid arthritis and osteoarthritis. RA is an autoimmune disorder when the body attacks its own cells, which often results in joint destruction. OA is wear-and-tear arthritis that comes with age or because of improper diet or lifestyle.

Cartilage, the joint lining, that acts as a shock absorber consists of water and collagen. Collagen matrix, the protein fibers that give cartilage its strength and shape, is insulated by a net that include glucosamine and chondroitin sulfate, two important building blocks, *that need vitamin D to work.*

Glucosamine is essential for production of water-binding proteins in cartilage, and chondroitin sulfates draw fluids that provide the ease of movement and attract nutrients for cartilage repair. Injury, wear, and corrosive enzymes can damage this protection, and cartilage loses the ability to repair itself. It gradually deteriorates and forms clefs and crevices that impede movement and cause pain.

The traditional approach to treating joint pain is well known – suppress the pain with aspirin, ibuprofen or other pain-killers. These drugs simply mask the problem by calming the symptoms while the joints keep deteriorating. Every pain-killing drug has a huge list of dangerous, long term effects. When you have them, they are not "side effects," they are *main* effects.

Luckily, there are other ways to deal with arthritis. Research shows that supplementing your body with two important cartilage building elements—glucosamine and chondroitin—can aid in joint restoration.

Another useful nutrient is MSM (methyl-sulfonyl-methane), a form of sulfur found in many common foods: fruits, vegetables, meat, fish and eggs. MSM helps to relieve pain and inflammation in joints and muscles. In addition, it boosts blood supply, lessens muscle spasms and softens scar tissue.

Cayenne pepper relieves arthritis pain

Capsicum, cayenne pepper extract *(yes, that hot spice!)*, was found by Dr. Christopher 50 years ago to help relieve arthritis pain and have many other uses, such as opening up your arteries to eliminate cold hands and feet. Cayenne opens up the circulatory system so that nutrients and oxygen can get to the joints experiencing pain. *Pain is the affected area's cry for more oxygen and more nutrients.* Avoid dairy products to avoid the calcification in the joints. Eating fresh healthy foods and mild exercise helps improve the circulation and speed up healing.

Lastly, your lifestyle and habits can help you avoid discomfort. Maintain your health, stay in shape and enjoying an active lifestyle will lower the risk of developing osteoarthritis. Osteoarthritis affects weight-bearing joints first. *If your joints have to manage extra weight, the cartilage is worn out faster than it can repair itself.*

The common belief is that osteoarthritis sufferers should not exercise, but research proves the opposite. Moderate exercise helps to keep joints healthy. Even if a person is already affected by arthritis, working the body helps stimulate the restoration process.

Here is a small exercise you can do to keep your knee joints in shape: bend your knees as if you were going to do a sit-up. Keeping your knees close together, move them in circular motions clockwise and then in the reverse direction.

You might not feel like moving when your arthritis flares up with burning pain, but a combination of diet, moderate exercise, supplements and topical preparations can prevent pain and allow you to enjoy your favorite activities. The real cause of arthritis is lack of vitamin D from the sun or in the diet from early age. We have become a nation of sun avoiders; more of us stay inside, shielded from its healing rays.

Vitamin D builds the immune system

Rheumatoid arthritis is an autoimmune disease. In this form of arthritis, the immune system attacks your own body *because it lacks vitamin D*, the hormone which directs the immune system to attack invading bacteria. Instead it goes crazy and attacks anything that it comes in contact with. This is the way AIDS and diabetes get started. The FDA has weighed in on this issue and says that preventing autoimmune diseases is one of the most important benefits of having adequate vitamin D in the body.

Here's what authorities from around the world say about vitamin D and arthritis.

Researchers from Harvard found that a supplement of 800 IU of D could reduce the risk of any type of fracture by 26%, whereas 400 IU did nothing. (If they would have used 4,000 IU, they might have found an almost complete elimination of fractures. Wouldn't that be a blessing!)

Drs. Feskanich and Willet found the consuming 800 IU or more of vitamin D reduced the risk of hip fracture by 37%, whereas adding milk or calcium supplement did nothing to reduce the risk of fracture. In fact, they actually increased the risk. This extensive study involved 72,000 women over a period of 18 years. The dairy lobby, you might imagine, does not like these results.

Dr. Merlino, lead investigator of the Iowa Women's Health Study, University of Iowa, studied 29,000 women for 11 years and found that those who consumed the most vitamin D were 33% less likely to have rheumatoid arthritis, and those that drank the least milk.

Dr. Arabelovic from Tufts-New England Medical Center, Division of Rheumatology in Boston, recommends the following treatment for arthritis: Optimize your weight, exercise, increase consumption of vitamins D and C, use creams and lotion for the pain and avoid long-term use of pain killers.

Dr. Cantorna from Penn State University reports that “increased vitamin D intakes might decrease the incidence and severity of autoimmune diseases and the rate of bone fracture.”

Dr. Glowacki of Brigham and Women's Hospital, Harvard Medical School, reports that women with arthritis often have osteoporosis. We already knew that, didn’t we?

off the mark
by Mark Parisi
PINEWOOD
ARTHRITIS
CARE CENTER
YOU JUST NEED TO FILL OUT A FEW FORMS FIRST...
10-11
www.offthemark.com
ATLANTIC FEATURE SYND. ©2000 MARK PARISI
MarkParisi@aol.com

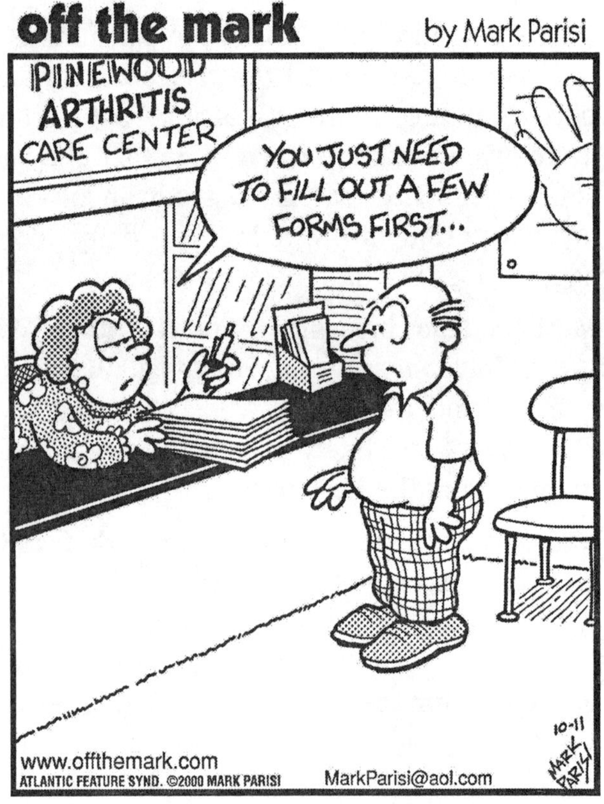

Cartoon copyrighted by Mark Parisi, printed with permission

Dr. Rennie of the MRC Human Nutrition Research, Cambridge, UK, reports that the use of pain killers, NSAIDS, and other drug therapies may increase the requirement for some nutrients such as vitamin D, zinc, calcium, folate and other B-vitamins. Also, Omega-3 may provide special benefits.

In Precrire International, researchers suggest that steroid therapy leads to loss of bone density. Some treatments may slow decline, but none have been shown to reverse decline, and the therapy that has the best risk-to-benefit-ratio is the use of vitamin D, magnesium, and calcium.

Dr. Miggiano GA, Centro di Ricerche in Nutrizione, Facolta di Medicina e Chirurgia, Universita Cattolica S.Cuore, Roma, Italia, emphasizes the importance of increasing Omega-3 fatty acids, antioxidants, folate, B-12, vitamins C and D in the diet. He also recommends limiting the use of steroids. Some people may also need to follow a diet that eliminates certain foods, like dairy products, to see if they are offensive to the patient.

Dr. Adams from Castle Medical Center in Hawaii reported that vitamin K could help prevent osteoporosis and deposition of calcium in the arteries which leads to heart disease. Eating five servings a day of fruit and vegetables generally provides sufficient vitamin K. Unfortunately many people only consume one serving or less per day.

Five tips to treat and manage arthritis

1. Dramatically increase vitamin D consumption from sun or fortified foods and consumption of vitamin C to 2,000 mg. per day
2. Use cayenne pepper to control pain and increase circulation
3. Avoid *all* dairy products for two weeks, then test to see if the pain is worse after dairy products are reintroduced
4. Exercise and stretch daily as much as possible without doing harm
5. Eat five servings a day each of fruits, vegetables and whole grains
6. Drink lots of water
7. Meditate every day using positive affirmations

For more detailed scientific information on this subject, go to www.vitaminDinfo.org

CHAPTER TWELVE

VITAMIN D AND CANCER

"Vitamin D deficiency has been associated with increased risks of deadly cancers, cardiovascular disease, multiple sclerosis, rheumatoid arthritis, and type I diabetes mellitus."

- Dr. Michael Holick
Boston University Medical Center

Cancer is a very tricky subject to deal with, so this chapter will discuss the findings of many scientific studies. While some of it may be difficult to follow, it will give you some insights on potentials for treating a disease so frightening to people. I've tried to make the information as basic and understandable as possible. If you are interested in reading the actual research, you will find it at the end of the chapter.

Vitamin D can lower cancer risk

High doses of vitamin D can reduce the risk of developing some common cancers by as much as 50%, US scientists claim. Researchers reviewed 63 old studies and found that the vitamin could reduce the chances of developing breast, ovarian and colon cancer, and others.

The research, done at the University of California in San Diego, looked at the relationship between blood levels of vitamin D and cancer risk. Survival rates for Afro-Caribbean people with breast, colon, prostate and ovarian cancers are worse than for caucasian people, possibly because dark skins are not as good at making vitamin D, the researchers said.

The papers reviewed, published worldwide between 1966 and 2004, included 30 investigations of colon cancer, 13 of breast cancer, 26 of prostate cancer and seven of ovarian cancer. Scientists said analysis showed that the vitamin D factor could not be ignored.

Taking 1,000 international units (IU) – or 25 micrograms – of the vitamin daily could lower an individual's cancer risk by 50% in colon cancer, and by 30% in breast and ovarian cancer, they said. Professor Cedric Garland, who led the review study, said “A preponderance of evidence, from the best observational studies the medical world has to offer...has led to the conclusion that public health action is needed.” In the absence of sunshine, a beneficial level of vitamin D could be obtained from a combination of food sources and supplements, he said.

Professor Garland warned that sun exposure had its own concerns. “Dark-skinned people, however, may need more exposure to produce adequate amounts of vitamin D, and some fair-skinned people shouldn’t try to get any vitamin D from the sun. The easiest and most reliable way of getting the appropriate amount is from food and a daily supplement.” The findings were published in the *American Journal of Public Health.*

FDA's point of view

Food and Drug Administration experts on vitamin D stated that "there is growing scientific evidence linking low circulating vitamin D to increased risk of osteoporosis, diabetes, cancer and autoimmune disorders." Their recommendation is that sufficient vitamin D should be supplied through dietary sources alone. It is evident from our review that vitamin D intake is often too low to sustain healthy circulating levels of 25-hydroxyvitamin D.

Officials at the FDA wouldn't say that the lack of vitamin D "leads to osteoporosis, diabetes, cancer and autoimmune disorders" if it wasn't true, now would they? I wouldn't and couldn't say that vitamin D is a cure-all for any chronic disease, but the FDA experts' opinion is very broad.

Huge database on cancer and D

The subject of vitamin D and cancer is so huge that I could not do it justice in 10 books, let alone, one chapter. With over 2,131 papers published on the topic already, and dozens more being published every week, Vitamin D research has become the primary focus at many universities. The best I can do is present the highlights. *For further information on the subject, log on to www.cholecalciferol-council.com.*

As I said earlier, vitamin D is essential to the form and function of every cell in the body. Evidently, when some cells don't get enough vitamin D they go wild and attack each other. The cells start growing uncontrollably, forming tumors and destroying their host.

Drug companies want monopoly control

Drug companies are feverishly trying to modify the vitamin D molecule to make it patentable. But so far, no variations are as safe and effective as good old natural D. Cancer-treating drugs are the most profitable drugs in the world and you would think there would be interest in natural, inexpensive and safe alternatives. With the evidence presented below, however, it will become clear that anyone who desperately wants to prevent or treat cancer should take a good hard look at combining vitamin D therapy with conventional treatments before being confined to a hospital bed and just maybe, you'll never have to go to a hospital. The hospital walk-out rate is not very high.

> *"A study of more than 3,100 veterans ages 50-75 who underwent screening colonoscopies found that subjects who consumed more than 645 IU per day of vitamin D were 40% less likely to have pre-cancerous colon polyps than those who got little or no vitamin D."*
>
> \- Journal of the American Medical Association
> December 10, 2003

Dr. Ed Giovannucci is an epidemiologist and a doctor from Harvard who has intensely studied the connection between the lack of sunshine for the body's production of vitamin D and cancer. His study shows that people with adequate levels of D in their blood have a 30% lower risk of developing *any* form of cancer. It's astounding that vitamin

D affects the development of every type of cancer. Thus, if people are going to treat any type of cancer, they should be sure to get adequate levels of D in their tissues. No patient in any hospital should be left without enough D in his or her body.

Dr. Chriatani at Harvard University found that vitamin D almost tripled the five year survival rate of patients with lung cancer. The five year survival rate was 72% in the group with the highest vitamin D intake compared to only 29% with the lowest. After this study was published you would think that every doctor in the country treating lung cancer would be recommending high doses of vitamin D to their cancer patients. But this just isn't happening.

Dr. Diane Feskanich and her coworkers at Harvard University found that women who had the highest plasma D levels had a 47% reduced risk of colon cancer.

Dr. Lowe from St. Goerges Medical School found that if women with certain genes were seven times more likely to get breast cancer, if they did not have at least 50nm/l of vitamin D in their plasma. This shows that people with certain genes need more vitamin D than others.

Dr. Hollis, Dr. Peters, and their coworkers at the National Cancer Institute found women with a certain gene were four times more likely to get colon cancer if their vitamin D levels were low. They found that added vitamin D reduced the risk of colon cancer by 73%.

Dr. Slattery at the University of Utah's Health Research Center found that women of a certain genotype could reduce their risk of rectal cancer by 48% with the most plasma D. Those that had the highest sun exposure reduced their risk by 41%. Impressive numbers!

Dr. Weitsman found that high vitamin D makes it easy for hydrogen peroxide to kill off breast cancer cells.

> *"Men who consumed higher levels of vitamin D reduced their overall cancer risk by at least 30 percent."*
>
> \- Ed Giovannucci
> Harvard researcher

Dr. Silverman from Cedars-Sinai Medical Center in Los Angeles found that women who had a fracture were much more likely to end up with additional fractures, heart attack and breast cancer. Evidently, low D is a major factor for all of these diseases.

Dr. Valrance of the University of Notre Dame found that high doses of vitamin D could reduce the risk of breast cancer for all females even if they had many relatives who had died of breast cancer.

Dr. Zhang wrote in the *Journal of Nutrition and Cancer* that milk consumption was strongly correlated with prostate cancer and breast cancer. Patients who avoided milk had 35% less risk of having either breast or prostate cancer.

Dr. Ganmaa of Japan found a close correlation between milk consumption and breast, ovarian, and uterine cancer because much of today's milk comes from pregnant cows.

Dr. Pritchard from Veterans Medical Center in Vermont found that patients with the highest plasma levels of D had 40%-50% less colon and rectum cancer, regardless of patient obesity and levels of fat and fiber in their diets.

Dr. Garland from the University of California-San Diego found a direct correlation between higher intensity of local sunshine and less breast cancer throughout the United States. He also found that areas of most sunshine had 60% less colon cancer.

Dr. Diaz from the School of Medical Sciences in Bristol, England, found that vitamin D would actually kill colon cancer cells. Dr. Thomas found that vitamin D would reduce the growth rate of colon cancer cells by 40%.

Dr. Berube from Quebec found that vitamin D could reduce breast densities, an indicator of later breast cancer.

CHAPTER THIRTEEN

HOW IMPORTANT IS D TO YOUR BRAIN?

"The number of Americans with dementia caused by Alzheimer's disease is expected to triple to 12 million by 2050. Yet the nation and its leaders have scarcely begun to consider the far-reaching implications of the aging of the U.S. population."

- President's Council on Bioethics report

The brain is a very complex organ. It's more complicated than the largest computer. Most of the time, it is self-repairing and self-regulating. It directs the manufacture of many compounds from the food you eat to make the millions of substances it needs to function healthfully. One of the things it needs and never seems to get enough of is vitamin D.

Vitamin D helps the brain produce serotonin – the feel-good neurotransmitter critical to emotional health. A deficiency can contribute to negative emotions such as depression. Conversely, increased vitamin D consumption elevates mood and promotes a positive outlook. Perhaps this is why people feel so good when they vacation in warm sunny places.

D deficiency rampant in mental health centers

According to vitamin expert John Cannell, MD, a California psychiatrist, vitamin D deficiency contributes to many mood problems. "About 90% of patients in my hospital are vitamin D deficient," he says, adding: "when I put them on a vitamin D regimen, it improves their mood disorders."

In particular, supplementation with vitamin D is known to prevent seasonal affected disorder (SAD). This nutrient is normally produced in the skin during exposure to sunlight, but as days grow shorter and colder in winter, the body is unable to produce adequate amounts of vitamin D. Individuals living at latitudes where the daylight hours shorten significantly, such as in the northern U.S., are most at risk for vitamin D deficiency and the resulting "winter depression." Clinical research shows that taking extra vitamin D during the winter can improve mood and ward off the wintertime blues. In a recent study covering 30 days of treatment comparing people receiving vitamin D supplementation with people who used light boxes for two hours a day, *depression completely resolved in the D group but not in the control group*.

In one double-blind trial, people received either 800 IU of vitamin D or a placebo for five days during late winter. Those taking vitamin D experienced a significant enhancement in positive mood compared to those taking the placebo. Particularly notable is the unusually rapid response produced by vitamin D supplementation. Individuals felt better after taking vitamin D for only five days.

Vitamin D supplement is essential

Of course, if you want to feel really good, it's best to supplement with vitamin D year-round, not just during the winter months. For people with limited sun exposure — housebound individuals, night-shift workers, women wearing robes and head coverings for religious purposes —

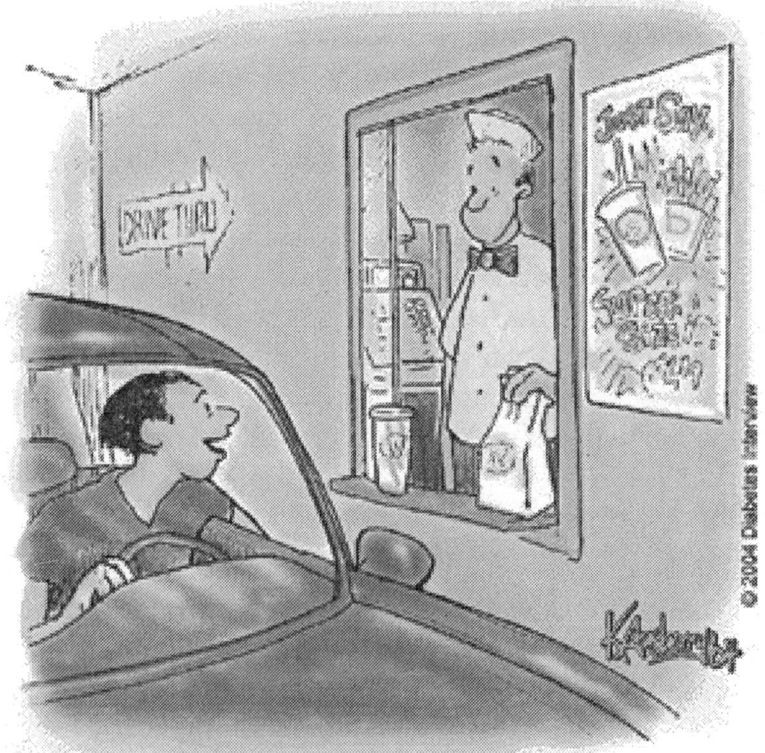

"...I was hoping you'd let me know how much more insulin I need to take if I decide to 'super-size' my order."

DIABETES HEALTH. PRINTED WITH PERMISSION.

daily Vitamin D supplementation is critical for maintaining emotional well-being. Moreover, vitamin D offers many other positive effects.

High stress may increase the need for vitamin D or UV-B sunlight, magnesium, and calcium. People with Parkinson's and Alzheimer's diseases have lower levels of vitamin D. Studies also show definite improvement if they also get a high-fiber, highly nutritional diet.

Nursing homes reject nutrition to maximize profits

I must tell you a story about a study we did in suburban Chicago at a nursing home for Alzheimer's patients. We put a study group on a daily diet of three slices of Natural Ovens Bakery's Whole Grain breads fortified with many nutrients, a tablespoon of Zesty Flax Energy Mix (an omega-3 supplement) and eight glasses of water (without ice) per day. Within six weeks, the people were more coherent and were feeling much better. Amazingly, the food also eliminated constipation and the patients were placed in a minimum care ward.

But when it came time to incorporate the food plan throughout the nursing home, the governing board said "absolutely not." The foods would have increased the home's costs by $1 a week per patient. Reportedly, the increase was too much, even though the nursing home was getting $1000 per week per patient for taking care of the patients and doing all that paper work. The epilogue to the story is that the nursing home feared they could lose money because it would no longer be paid for constipation treatments and received less money for the residents who had been moved into lower cost units. Penny wise and pound foolish at the cost of depriving our elderly the comfort and functionality they deserve.

Drugs increase need for D

Dr. Drezner from the University of Wisconsin found that anti-convulsing drugs induce osteoporosis and many bone problems. He recommends that all patients on anti-epileptic drugs automatically be given at least 2,000 IU of vitamin D per day plus 600 mg. of calcium. Doses of 15,000 IU per day may be needed for those with muscle-bone pain. She does not recommend the use of Fosamax™ for such patients. I would also recommend foods that are fortified with magnesium, folic acid, B-6 and B-12.

Dr. Jekovee-Vrhovsek in Slovenia found that children with cerebral palsy need high doses of vitamin D and some calcium to prevent bone loss. This is probably true for all bed-ridden patients and others forced to stay indoors most of the time.

CHAPTER FOURTEEN

VITAMIN D HELPS YOU BREATHE EASIER

> *"Probably 40 percent of otherwise healthy adults between 49 and 65 years old and half of all people over 65 are deficient."*
>
> \- Dr. Michael Holick
> Boston University Medical Center

A major, newly-released study of 14,000 U.S. residents shows that those with the most vitamin D in their blood have much better lung capacity than those with the least. As most people age, their breathing capacity diminishes and when death is eminent, breathing capacity is near zero. So breathing capacity has a lot to do with how young you feel and how old you really are, regardless of what the calendar says. People have long attributed lung capacity to exercise, but now it also seems to depend on how much vitamin D you are absorbing from the sun while you are exercising. Heart capacity, another indicator of not aging, is also related to vitamin D levels.

This from a Science News article by Janet Raloff:

D increases Lung Capacity

"Peter Black, an internist from the University of Auckland, New Zealand, found many people can't breathe well because of emphysema and chronic bronchitis. Many smokers have these problems. Evidently, vitamin D helps prevent these problems.

Black told *Science News Online*, 'We were taken aback at how large the effect was.' The study showed that people who never smoked but who were getting little vitamin D had 35 percent worse lung function than did former smokers who were getting adequate amounts of the vitamin. Current smokers, regardless of their vitamin D intake, had worse lung function than did either of these groups.

"For their study, Black and Scragg grouped the participants into five roughly equal-size groups on the basis of how much vitamin D was in their blood. The group with the lowest D had no more than 40 nanomoles of the vitamin per liter (nmol/l) of blood, whereas the group with the highest concentration had at least 85 nmol/l. However, Black notes, the effect of vitamin D on lung function is larger than what other studies have attributed to eating diets rich in fruits and antioxidant vitamins or to most environmental factors other than smoking.

"Indeed, people with too little vitamin D appear to be paying a toll in health status, according to a trio of researchers from Boston University School of Medicine, the University of California and the San Francisco-based Sunlight, Nutrition and Health Research Center. Their new analysis, reported in the November *Photochemistry and Photobiology*, looked at U.S. incidences of diseases that appear to be higher in people with low vitamin D-blood concentrations from osteoporosis-linked fractures to certain cancers. Overall, the researchers calculate, as many as 50,000 people may die prematurely in the United States each year from diseases related to vitamin D deficiency, at an estimated cost to society of at least $40 billion. That's at least seven times as much as the annual U.S. cost of cataracts and skin cancers attributable to possible excess sun exposure. There is virtually no evidence that sensible sun exposure increases skin cancer risk."

50,000 deaths a year at a cost to taxpayers of $40 billion is an awfully high price to pay for avoiding the sun and not taking enough D. We need to do something about this lack of adequate vitamin D. If you have an idea, contact me at info.vitaminDinfo.org.

CHAPTER FIFTEEN

HOW MUCH D DO YOU NEED?

"Vitamin D helps all of womankind."

- Paul Stitt, M.S., Biochemist

Daily deficiency of Vitamin D is killing many Americans. The slow response of the Food and Nutrition Board's recommendation to raise the intake level of vitamin D is literally destroying people and committing them to a life of pain and suffering. The Food and Nutrition Board is a quasi-public organization designed to make recommendations to the FDA on nutritional requirements. It appears the FNB is made up of individuals who are working in the best interests of the drug industry, not the American public.

Food and Nutrition Board ignores scientific proof

At the last hearing on setting vitamin D intake levels, the board invited and heard testimony from two prominent U.S. vitamin D researchers. The FNB totally ignored their presentation and set the recommended intake level on non-existent research. There are literally hundreds of people doing research on vitamin D in this country and virtually every one of them say that the present level is set ridiculously low, but the FNB continues to ignore them. Thus far, the FDA has refused to step in and reset the level of vitamin D in agreement with present information from peer-reviewed scientific reports.

If an average person adds 1,000 IU of D3 to his or her diet, a significant rise in serum blood levels will be noted. Any lower dose has an insignificant effect. However, most scientists say the level needs to be raised to 100nmol/l. In order for an average person to attain this, the intake would need to be about 5,000 IU per day based on our research and that of others.

None of us is "average"

The word "average" is misleading. If you have been on a diet that is deficient in vitamin D, you may need to take 10,000 IU per day for three months just to catch up. We know that people who use legally prescribed drugs need to take in much more vitamin D because many drugs interfere with the action of activating vitamin D in the body. Also, if people are obese, they need more because vitamin D is fat soluble and gets dispersed throughout the fat tissues. Thus, overweight people need to have their blood levels of vitamin D checked to see if they have enough to be healthy. Also people who stay indoors or wear lots of clothes when they are out-of-doors need more vitamin D. In winter in the northern states, *nobody* gets the direct sunshine needed. People over 65 also need more since they, as a group, seem to be slow metabolizers. This probably includes most of the people living in the US. The present recommended intake covers none of these people.

Current RDA level set in 1940s

The present RDA was set in the *1940s* and we're still stuck with it. Since then, 38,000 articles have been published about vitamin D. These articles are housed in the National Library of Medicine and are purposefully being ignored by the Institute of Medicine. Is it because it might impair the profits of the medical industry? They set the dietary level at 400 IU based on the fact that babies who received that dosage from cod liver oil did not get rickets. It has not been increased to recognize the fact that *adults are larger than babies and the fact that vitamin D deficiency has now been linked to about 50 different undesirable conditions.* (I refuse to call them diseases because they are *conditions caused by nutritional deficiency*). These conditions should never be treated by prescribed drugs because they are *nutritional deficiencies, not drug deficiencies. However, it is a lot more profitable to treat them with drugs.*

Based on the latest peer-reviewed scientific literature, the list includes nearly all maladies known to mankind, because vitamin D affects the form and function of every cell in our body, including skin cells, liver cells, kidney cells, heart cells, pancreas cells, fat cells, bone cells, muscle cells and brain cells. When these cells malfunction, we call it osteoporosis, arthritis, chronic pain, cancer, diabetes, heart disease, fibromyalgia, depression, hyperactivity or autoimmune disease. Getting adequate amounts of D into every cell helps these cells to function normally so that many of these "diseases" disappear; proving that *they were not real diseases, but simply nutrient deficiencies.*

Don't be conservative about your own health

With tons of research showing that vitamin D bolsters muscle and bone strength, improves insulin action, builds strong immunity against a multitude of diseases, and prevents many chronic disease, it begs the question: "How much vitamin D is enough?" Vitamin D has a *big* job to do. If you have health issues, this is not the time to be conservative.

On the toxic side, we know for sure *that a million units a day is probably toxic;* 40,000 is on the high side, but not dangerous to most people, and *600 is just not nearly enough.* This wide range, 600-40,000 makes the decision a lot easier. Low inputs of D are harming billions of the world's people, while *only two people have been harmed* (not killed) *by an overdose* by ingesting over a million IU daily, according to the scientific literature.

Take charge of your life

You can make a decision for yourself about how much to take. Try it for three months; note what you experience and then change the amount, if you like. This is probably the best way to find your own *personal* Fountain of Youth. We do know that some people need much more than others and some people have different ideas of what constitutes "good health."

First off, people with naturally darker skin pigmentation – Spanish, Italian, and African-American, for example – need 2-50 times as much sun exposure as a person with pale skin exposed to the bright noonday sun, according to Dr. Holick.

Experts agree: raise vitamin D levels

Last year, in a roundtable discussion at an osteoporosis conference in Lausanne, Switzerland, Drs. Vieth, Holick, Heaney, and others agreed that an optimal 25-D blood concentration for most people is 75 to 80 nmol/l. Therefore, have your blood checked for 25 Hydroxy D and try to maintain a level of at least 100 nmol/l (about 5,000 IU daily). Dr. Vieth is holding his own serum level at 300 nmol/l with 8,000 IU per day.

In people over the age of 60, vitamin D blood concentrations correlate with leg strength, according to studies by Bess Dawson-Hughes and her colleagues at the Agriculture Department's Human Nutrition Research Center on Aging in Boston. In one study, they examined data from 4,100 adults representing a cross-section of the U.S. population. People with vitamin D concentrations of 40 nmol/l or less walked more slowly and had more trouble rising from a chair than did people with concentrations higher than 86 nmol/l. The results took into account differences between the groups in age, arthritis, weight and use of a cane, according to the report in the *American Journal of Clinical Nutrition.*

You deserve optimal, not minimal health

Few people have the blood concentrations of vitamin D that researchers recommend. For instance, Hanley, at the Experimental Biology meeting in Washington, D.C., described a study of 200 Calgary adults. A third of the study's population showed less than 30 nmol/l during at least part of the year. "The average level of vitamin D through the four seasons was in the low 60s [nmol/l]," Hanley told *Science News*. If 80 nmol/l is taken as the cutoff for adequate vitamin D, "virtually 100% of the population is vitamin D deficient at least part of the year," he says.

Dr. Vieth says that "published cases of vitamin D toxicity with hypercalcemia, for which the vitamin D concentration and vitamin D dose are known, all involve intake of *more* than 40,000 IU per day."

FDA weighs in on deficiency

In the March, 2003, *Nutrition Reviews*, Mona Calvo of the U.S. Food and Drug Administration, co-authored a review of five studies on vitamin D status in Canada and the United States. She described data indicating a high incidence of vitamin D *insufficiency* in almost all populations. She also reported that *excess phosphate* interferes with the process of building bone. She found that most meat and milk products – especially processed meats and cheese – are excessively high in phosphate. Perhaps, this is why heavy dairy users have no more vitamin D in their blood than people who drink *no* cow's milk. Dr. Walt Willet from Harvard found that heavy dairy product users actually have more fractures than people who do not use milk products. Scientific articles published by the dairy industry cannot always be believed.

Read one book...stop heart disease

If you are suffering from heart disease and from the many drugs with horrible side effects used by the medical industry, I wrote just the book for you. It's called *The Real Cause of Heart Disease is not Cholesterol.* It tells you just how to tame the cholesterol monster and reduce your chances by over 90% of dying prematurely (before age 90). It puts you in control of your future. For help in doing this in the kitchen, check out the *Natural Ovens Cookbook.* Both books are available by calling 800-772-0730.

What's the remedy?

Some researchers propose that fortified foods can cover vitamin D shortfalls. However, the current standard American diet offers, *at most,* 200-400 IU per day. Furthermore, Dr. Calvo has new data showing that "African-Americans do not consume [vitamin-D] fortified milk" – fortified with only 100 IU per 8 ounces. She suspects that many avoid milk because they have difficulty digesting it. To get enough D from milk one would need to drink 40 glasses a day (or eat three pounds of liver or two pounds of fatty fish every day).

Harold L. Newmark of Rutgers University in New Brunswick, N.J., and his colleagues proposed a new food-enrichment scheme in the Aug. 1, 2005, *American Journal of Clinical Nutrition*. They argue that the best way to help vulnerable groups get enough vitamin D would be to mandate fortification of grain-based products, such as wheat flour, corn meal and pasta.

Dr. John Cannell, the unpaid volunteer who keeps up the fabulous *www.cholecalciferol-council.com* website says:

"The IOM's Food and Nutrition Board issued their guidelines in 1997. Although over eight years old, the guidelines still have powerful effects on both practicing physicians and clinical researchers. The *guidelines used* not only recommend *absurdly inadequate daily intake levels*, they *erroneously* state that 2,000 units of vitamin D are potentially toxic. Research in the last five years shows just the opposite! If fact, healthy humans utilize about 4,000 units of vitamin D a day. Some of us get it from the sun in the summer, but many people avoid the sun and *get less* than 1,000 units a day."

4,000 IU per day is safe and effective

Dr. Vieth states that the "4,000 IU daily dosage of vitamin D3 effectively increased the vitamin D levels to high-normal concentrations in practically all adults and the serum 25(OH)D remained within the physiologic range; therefore, we consider 4,000 IU vitamin D3 per day to be a very safe intake."

Your future health is up to you. Please question doctors who prescribe more than 1,000 mg. of calcium a day – in addition to what you are already getting from your vegetables and other foods or supplements – because too much calcium interferes with activation of vitamin D and can be toxic and create calcification in soft tissues like your arteries and muscles.

Watch out for excess calcium

When we say "high calcium is a danger" what we really mean is that a diet high in calcium and protein and phosphate is hazardous to your health. Excess phosphate binds with the calcium to make it insoluble and high animal protein foods tend to be high in phosphate. Here, excesses are the problem. Moderation is the key.

Let's take a look at cow's milk products. Cow's milk is much higher in calcium than human milk, and if you are reading this book, you are probably weaned from your mother. In less developed countries in this world that has much less osteoporosis and arthritis than Americans, the RDA for calcium is about 500 mg. per day. Isn't that amazing? Of course, they get much more sun than most Americans.

There are some foods that speed up the aging process, like cow's milk and refined and processed foods. Cow's milk is perfectly designed to feed a baby calf and speed up its growing and aging process. A baby calf needs to grow up fast, gaining 600 pounds in one year, to be able to defend itself. But, as humans growing beyond our youthful years, we should think about *slowing down* the aging process.

The Fountain of Youth

Yes, I do believe that vitamin D is an important part of the fountain of youth. Scientifically speaking, no other vitamin or drug has been shown to be able to do as much to alleviate human suffering as adding vitamin D at adequate levels to every person's diet.

Since having been on a 10,000 IU of D per day diet myself for six months, not only are my muscles stronger, my hair has started growing in darker roots which has amazed and surprised me and my friends. My ability and desire to exercise has dramatically increased. I am truly convinced that what the scientific literature says about the many benefits of vitamin D is really true. I like ideas that are scientifically valid and work for me personally.

In my 40 years of intensively studying nutrition, I have learned that all nutrients must be available and work together synergistically to provide a "Fountain of Youth." I have also learned to avoid dairy products, foods that contain hydrogenated fats, white flour, sugar and any kind of corn syrup.

I have found that a Chinese herbal tonic that contains 18 different herbs, called JC Tonic. *(To obtain information on the JCTonic – www.jurak.com ID#12584 or call toll free: 1-866-448-5796, ID#12584)*. JC Tonic can be of huge benefit when combined with a D-rich diet to someone seeking the fountain of youth. I can't imagine living without at least five servings each per day of fresh vegetables, fresh fruits, whole grains, legumes, seeds & nuts, filtered water, exercise, the JC Tonic, vitamin D-fortified dark chocolates and perhaps a little wine. Because of the chewing action, the digestive enzymes mix in with the food and allow the D and other nutrients to be best utilized at the cellular level. It is far better to get your nutrients from fortified foods than it is from pills that may be poorly digested. To me, eating healthy, chewy food is an everyday part of the enjoyment of living.

Vitamin D info needs lots of promotion

Vitamin D knowledge is something that most health writers, doctors and dietitians have overlooked until very recently. Our ancestors were sun worshippers and I have become one now and totally enjoying at least 20–30 minutes in the direct sun daily when we are in warm climates. I love being out in the sun but never take it to the extreme point of burning my skin, and I still eat vitamin D-fortified breads, cookies, chocolates and drink mixes every day just to be sure.

> *"Women fare worse than men because they abruptly lose bone-protecting estrogen at menopause. Nursing homes are full of hunched, shrunken grandmas, hobbling behind walkers after being admitted solely because of a broken hip."*
>
> \- Bernadine Healy, M.D.
> On Health

In January, 2005, my wife and I "retired" from management of our original company and began a new company developing a line of super healthy foods that people *really* love to eat, dark chocolate! This is a high risk adventure. First, we have to educate people about how badly they need vitamin D and a healthy lifestyle by getting the media involved. We can't do it without the media. Secondly, the labeling restrictions on making a healthy food or dietary supplement are unbelievable.

December, 2005

Dear Mr. Stitt:

I am 93 years old. I am on a dozen medications. I have not been able to walk without a walker since I fell 5 years ago. I have been on vitamin D rich dark chocolates for 2 months now. I feel a lot better and much stronger. I can move much faster, and I do many more things around the house. The chocolates satisfy my cravings, and seem to reduce my appetite, but don't have a funny aftertaste like a lot of other chocolates. I am looking forward to doing my gardening in the spring. Thank God for these chocolates.

Sincerely,

Phyllis

One might suspect there's a faction that wants to make it almost impossible to tell the customer the truth about how much they will benefit from healthy food. Then, to survive in the marketplace, you have to keep the customers happy, the stores happy, and the bankers behind you. Luckily, we are retired and don't really need to make more money to be happy. Seeing people get well and write to us about it and share their success with others gives us so much happiness. If you want to be in our next book, tell us about your results.

Make yourself happy!

We are still working to make foods that are loaded with antioxidants, vitamin C and E, folate, B-6, B-12, calcium, magnesium, selenium and chromium to make the 1,500 to 2,000 IU of vitamin D in each cluster of the dark chocolates maximally effective. Our new venture may be the first company in the United States to produce and market such products. It will take a lot of God's blessing and many strong supporters to make it successful. For more information about these products, go to *www.healthychocolate-treats.com.*

DRUG-FREE AMERICA
HISTORY OF SOMEONE BORN BEFORE I WAS
12 MILLION LAYOFFS
GRIND
AGE 0-4
AMOXICILLIN
4-12
RITALIN
12-18
APPETITE SUPPRESSANTS
18-24
NO-DOZ
24-38
PROZAC
38-65
ZANTAC
65—
EVERYTHING ELSE

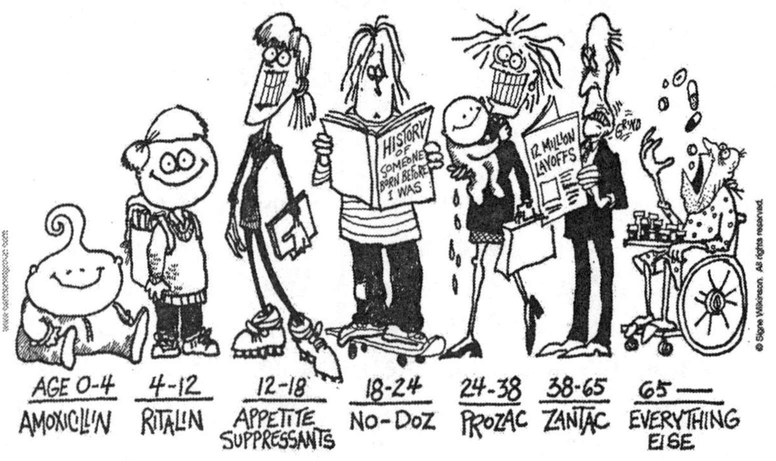

Cartoon copyrighted by Signe Wilkinson. Printed with permission.

To recap, how to achieve your own **Fountain of Youth** is really pretty basic. Dedicate some time to yourself to learn about how best to take care of your body. No one can do this as well for you as yourself.

1. Get 4,000 to 5,000 IU of vitamin D every day from several sources.

2. Eat five servings a day each of fresh fruit, vegetables and whole grain breads made with flax.

3. Drink lots of water – eight glasses each day. The size of the glass depends on the size of your body.

4. Get some exercise every day, preferably outside. Sweat a little!

5. Take an herbal tonic every day.

6. Avoid hydrogenated fats, corn syrup and white flour.

7. Maintain a healthy spirit.

8. Be happy – greet everyone with a big smile.

May all of your days
be blessed
with good health
and longevity...
and let there
be light
in your quest
for knowledge!

EPILOGUE

WANT TO CUT HEALTH CARE COSTS?

PRACTICE "P" BEFORE "T" WITH "D"

"The pharmaceutical industry promises health and promises cures, and yet what it delivers is a lifetime of continued disease and dependence on profit-building pharmaceuticals."

- Dr. Matthias Rath,
Dr. Rath Foundation

We hear a lot of shouting about spiraling medical care costs and the growing number of families unable to afford insurance, but few people and fewer politicians even whisper the "P" word. Not our politicians who warn of darker days ahead. Not business that struggles to pay the costs. Nor medical professionals who are in the very best position to bring relief to ailing Americans and their pocketbooks.

The P word stands for disease PREVENTION. It's a very small "p" in the medical profession's lexicon and barely exists in the pharmaceutical industry where the cash cow is Treatment with a capital "T". Cynics even speculate that the drug industry's long-term profitability is dependent upon keeping generation after generation of Americans sick and popping lots of pills.

How serious is the problem? Let's review, for example, the cost of falls and fractures where I live in one small county of just 80,000 people, Manitowoc County, Wisconsin. Each year falls and fractures cost us more than $12 million. Then add an estimated $60 million for nursing home care after hospitalization, according to the County Health Center. That equates to $900 per year *per citizen* of Manitowoc County. And there's also the cost of suffering of our elderly who heal slowly. About 20% of older citizens who have a major fall die within the first year. Nationally, medical costs are about $1.7 *trillion.*

Incredibly, prevention is simple and inexpensive. There are hundreds of scientific studies showing that vitamin D deficiency is the major cause of falls, fractures, chronic pain, osteoporosis and many other afflictions. It's estimated that 96% of those over age 50 and 90% of females over age 20 are vitamin D deficient. The Mayo Clinic itself reported that 93% of its fracture patients are deficient. The good news: researchers predict that the rate of falls and fractures could be cut in half in 3-6 months if Americans consumed enough vitamin D. And that's the problem.

The best source of vitamin D is sunlight. However, an adequate level of absorption requires exposing at least 30% of bare skin for at least 30 minutes a day, not possible for those of us living in the northern latitudes from November through March. And during the summer, an exaggerated concern over skin cancer induces people to lather up with sunblock that prevents vitamin D absorption, but allows penetration of harmful rays. Ironically, vitamin D helps *prevent* the most deadly forms of skin cancer.

Vitamin D from food? Studies of fortified milk samples show a wide variance and inadequate levels. Fatty fish is rich in D but you have to eat the fat that may also contain mercury. Remember the cod liver oil our mothers would force upon us? A full tablespoon a day still helps, but doesn't taste very good. You can, however, get enough vitamin D by eating five pounds of liver and 50 eggs, and fortunately a few food companies carefully enrich their products with adequate levels. You need to read the nutrition labels.

There's also the question of what's an adequate daily level. Decades ago, the FDA arbitrarily set 400 units per day as the recommended level, just enough to prevent rickets in *children*. That level is wholly inadequate for growing strong bones and joints, for post-menopausal women and dangerously low for seniors. Scientific literature reports that 2,000 units per day is perfectly safe and, if deficient, as much as 10,000 units per day may be required for some people.

So why aren't the drug companies pushing vitamin D like all those pain-killers they spend millions marketing that, in effect, only mask the causes of pain. Vitamin D is not patentable and very cheap to produce. Money is to be made in *relieving pain*, not eliminating it. And sadly, most of those pain-killers create side effects, some painful, that require another drug, and then another drug to mask the effects. Read the warning labels. *Vitamin D gives only beneficial effects*. Researchers continue to be amazed at just how necessary vitamin D is to preventing a widening range of maladies. Scientific studies have shown that adequate vitamin D and improving lifestyle can cut falls and fractures by 49%, heart disease by 25%, diabetes by 25%, arthritis by 40% and cancer by 30%. Plus, adequate vitamin D and improving diet, as we suggest, and exercising, can extend your life by adding nine happy years to your life, not more years of suffering.

By fortifying more foods with adequate levels of vitamin D and making it available as a dietary supplement, it's estimated that the nation could cut its medical bill by nearly 30%, saving $510 billion per year. Cost of providing the vitamin would be about 50 cents per person per day, totaling perhaps $50.3 billion, less than a tenth of the cost we now pay for medical care. Adding what could be saved in Medicare, Medicaid and by insurance companies and out-of-pocket expenses could bring the annual total *savings to $460 billion!* This could balance the U.S. budget and help reduce our national debt!

So what can we do? We can encourage our physicians to become better informed about good nutrition; especially about the benefits of vitamin D. Testing patients for vitamin D levels would provide the first clue in diagnosing a wide range of maladies. Businesses can help by educating their employees about the importance of vitamin D. As consumers, we can make reading nutrition labels on food packages a regular habit. And for our growing elderly population, our hospitals and nursing homes can start administering 2,000 units of vitamin D daily. There's ample scientific evidence that doing so will relieve pain and make their golden years safer, more comfortable and more enjoyable.

Want to cut our health care costs? Start prevention with the help of vitamin D to avoid expensive treatment. Simple, inexpensive and good business.

ADDDITIONAL BOOKS AVAILABLE THROUGH NATURAL PRESS

For more information or to order, call 800-772-0730

KEEPING IT OFF

Weight Loss Success Stories from those who did it!

by Barbara Stitt, Ph.D. & Melissa Luedtke

A collection of letters from real people who have taken the weight off and kept it off, and their tips to success.

Paperback; 153 pages

THE REAL CAUSE OF HEART DISEASE IS NOT CHOLESTEROL

by Paul A. Stitt M.S., C.N.S.

Stop heart disease in its tracks! Right now, 62 million people are heading straight toward cardiac failure. For most of them the danger can be averted; not with drugs, not with surgery – with KNOWLEDGE. Recent scientific research holds the key to discovering a whole new approach to heart health, an approach that the conventional medical community ignores: nutritional therapy. Learn inside how you can take control and maximize the quality of life, the WE-FOBAM way.

Paperback; 203 pages

THE NATURAL OVENS COOKBOOK

A collection of over 150 recipes from our customer's family kitchens and our test kitchen. Half of the recipes can be served in less than 60 minutes.

FOOD AND BEHAVIOR

by Barbara Reed Stitt

Can what people eat really affect the way they behave? The evidence says yes! In this book, Barbara Reed Stitt, a former Chief Probation Officer and creator of a nutritional program which has helped thousands to lead healthy and productive lives, shows the link between food and behavior.

The connection between food and behavior is so basic that it is being overlooked by parents, the school system, counselors and most of the medical professionals. Ask any hyperactive child, depressed, angry teenager, violent adult or criminal what they eat and you'll find they "live" on junk food – sweetened boxed cereals, candy, carbonated drinks, potato chips, fast foods. Junk food abuses the mind, under-nourishes the body and distorts behavior.

Food & Behavior is a book for people in trouble with their health and behavior – and for all of you who don't want members of your family to get in trouble. Barbara's message is both enlightening and encouraging.

Paperback; 223 pages

BEATING THE FOOD GIANTS

by Paul A. Stitt

Paul Stitt, a biochemist whose outspoken criticism of the American food industry has won him national attention now reveals the processes by which the food giants determine what you eat...and HOW MUCH you eat!

Paul Stitt draws on his years as a food scientist for two of the country's largest corporations, and lays bare the greed and the cover-ups taking place in board rooms and laboratories across the nation!

Paperback, 300 pages

WHY GEORGE SHOULD EAT BROCCOLI

by Paul A. Stitt

Did you know that...

– special foods can provide athletes with more endurance, faster recovery, and prevent sore muscles?

– there are over 900 compounds in whole foods that can prevent cancer and other degenerative diseases such as arthritis, heart disease, and diabetes?

– broccoli, just one vegetable, has 33 compounds that help prevent the development of tumors?

Paperback; 399 pages

WHY CALORIES DON'T COUNT

by Paul A. Stitt

Did you know...

– calorie counting is highly inacurate?

– a low-calorie diet can make you sick, irritable and even cause emotional illness?

– you can eat more than you're eating now and still be slimmer?

– stopping a food addiction may solve your weight problem?

Paul Stitt, M.S., will show you how to satisfy the body's hunger with a minimum of calories and will tell you about the neglected nutrient which will let you eat MORE and lose weight!

So if you're tired of the dieting routine, if you want to slim down and stay slim and never be hungry again, don't "weight" another minute! Read "Why Calories Don't Count"!

Paperback; 219 pages